Coping with Mild Cognitive Impairment (MCI)

of related interest

**Dementia – Support for Family and
Friends, Second Edition**
Dave Pulsford and Rachel Thompson
ISBN 978 1 78592 437 8
eISBN 978 1 78450 811 1

**A Pocket Guide to Understanding Alzheimer's
Disease and Other Dementias, Second Edition**
Dr James Warner and Dr Nori Graham
ISBN 978 1 78592 458 3
eISBN 978 1 78450 835 7

**Reducing the Symptoms of Alzheimer's
Disease and Other Dementias**
A Guide to Personal Cognitive Rehabilitation Techniques
Jackie Pool
ISBN 978 1 78592 578 8
eISBN 978 1 78450 992 7

Will I Still Be Me?
**Finding a Continuing Sense of Self in the
Lived Experience of Dementia**
Christine Bryden
ISBN 978 1 78592 555 9
eISBN 978 1 78450 950 7

What the Hell Happened to My Brain?
Living Beyond Dementia
Kate Swaffer
ISBN 978 1 84905 608 3
eISBN 978 1 78450 073 3

COPING WITH MILD COGNITIVE IMPAIRMENT (MCI)

A Guide to Managing Memory
Loss, Effective Brain Training and
Reducing the Risk of Dementia

MARY JORDAN

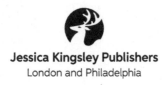

Jessica Kingsley Publishers
London and Philadelphia

The information contained in this book is not intended to replace the services of trained medical professionals or to be a substitute for medical advice. You are advised to consult a doctor on any matters relating to your health, and in particular on any matters that may require diagnosis or medical attention.

First published in 2020
by Jessica Kingsley Publishers
73 Collier Street
London N1 9BE, UK
and
400 Market Street, Suite 400
Philadelphia, PA 19106, USA

www.jkp.com

Copyright © Mary Jordan 2020

Front cover image source: Shutterstock.

Library of Congress Cataloging in Publication Data
A CIP catalog record for this book is available from the Library of Congress

British Library Cataloguing in Publication Data
A CIP catalogue record for this book is available from the British Library

ISBN 978 1 78775 090 6
eISBN 978 1 78775 091 3

Printed and bound in Great Britain

Contents

Chapter 1

What Is Mild Cognitive Impairment (MCI)?

Mild cognitive impairment (MCI) is considered to be simply a descriptive term for impaired memory or slight impairments in other areas of brain function such as planning or attention span. In some countries 'cognitive impairment' is used instead of the term 'dementia' to refer to a specific diagnosis where there is a memory problem and evidence of brain atrophy. In the UK the term 'dementia' would be used to describe this and so, in this book it is reserved to refer to this condition.

Dementia is not the same as MCI. Because it is not a disease or a medical condition, strictly speaking, you cannot have a 'diagnosis' of MCI. At the present time in the UK, MCI is not considered to be a medical condition or disease.

People who have MCI may take longer to do tasks or to plan and order a major action, but they do not experience significant problems in carrying out the functions of everyday living.

What does the term 'functions of everyday living' mean? It simply means the things you have to do to carry on your daily life – such as washing, dressing, preparing a meal, doing the shopping and so on, and also includes more complicated things like managing finances or planning a holiday. People who have MCI are still able to do all these things and are capable of living alone independently and managing ordinary everyday activities. They may take more time than others to come to a decision or take longer to plan and carry out actions, but they are not unable to manage these functions of everyday living.

Someone with MCI may have some difficulties with planning something like a social event or an outing, and may take longer to organize it. It can also be more difficult for someone with MCI to plan for the future – for example, to think about changing electricity supplier or moving money into a different savings account. This doesn't mean that someone with MCI is unable to do these things – it is simply that it may be more difficult for them to do so or it may take them a bit longer to arrange. People with MCI may also have more difficulty recalling things like the names of people, places or items, but given time, and when not under stress, they will likely be able to manage recall, perhaps with some reminders.

MCI can be defined as cognitive impairment, especially short-term memory loss which is beyond what would be expected given age and level of education but which is not significant enough to interfere with the activities of everyday living.

MCI is not just to do with getting old. This is important because memory problems, confusion and attention difficulties are often simply written off as problems of ageing. Many of us take longer to do things as we age, we think more slowly, we move more slowly and (perhaps due to frailty) we may be unable to complete some actions. But look again at the above definition: MCI is cognitive impairment that is considered to be *beyond what would be expected given age and level of education*. Being less agile and thinking more slowly may be 'age-related', meaning that this is what we might expect of an older person, but taken alone, these conditions are *not* evidence of MCI.

This book is not supposed to replace medical advice; if you are worried that you are developing dementia, please consult your doctor. They may then refer you for further investigations. If, eventually, you are diagnosed with some form of dementia, help and support is available.[1]

There is genuine confusion amongst non-medically trained people with respect to the difference between dementia and MCI, and so the following information should help distinguish between the two conditions.

Is it dementia?

People who have dementia will have a noticeable decline in communication, learning, remembering and problem-solving. This decline may occur very slowly over time and so the symptoms may be noticed first by a friend or relative who has not been in contact for a while.

These are the sorts of symptoms that occur with dementia:

- *Short-term memory loss*: this means forgetting something that was said or done within a few minutes. The first indication may be often-repeated questions to which the answers have already been supplied. For example, 'Where are we going this morning?' Sometimes an observer may notice that 'stories' are constantly repeated and the speaker has no recollection of having told the story even a few minutes before.

- *Impaired judgement*: this can mean something like perhaps taking risks when driving or trying to carry out a task clearly beyond the person's ability. People who do not have dementia may be stubborn if advised not to undertake an activity, but they would usually recognize that the advice given is correct. Someone who has dementia may not even understand that they are taking a risk or attempting something beyond their abilities.

- *Difficulties with abstract thinking*, such as being unable to plan for a future occasion – organizing a holiday, for example: this can sometimes be masked by the person with cognitive problems simply agreeing with whatever is suggested. Relatives may just think that the person in question has become more passive or less contentious. Sometimes the person who has this problem will 'put off' taking actions or making plans and suggest that they will 'do it tomorrow' or perhaps tell you that they are 'too tired' to tackle the task at this particular moment. Indeed, unusual procrastination can be one of the first signs to make relatives think something is wrong.

- *Faulty reasoning*: this is using illogical arguments to make a point or suggesting that something has happened that is highly unlikely. A common symptom is the mislaying of an item such as a purse or set of keys. When the item is found (after an extensive search) in a strange place (under the bed is a common example), the person with dementia will claim that they had nothing to do with the loss and suggest that 'someone' has deliberately hidden the item. This kind of illogical argument might be used even if the person lives alone and no one else has access to their belongings.
- *Inappropriate behaviour*, such as walking to the head of a queue rather than waiting in turn, interrupting a conversation, choosing to go out in unpleasant weather, and wearing clothes unsuited to the occasion or climate.
- *Loss of communication skills*: this can take many forms such as difficulty in expressing a point, losing the thread of a sentence, needing simplified answers to questions or failure to initiate conversation.
- *Disorientation to time and place*, such as losing the way in familiar surroundings, getting up and dressed during the night without reason, or going to bed at inappropriate times.
- *Gait, motor and balance problems*: this is not a common symptom but can manifest with some forms of dementia; a 'shuffling' walk may be present or unexplained falls may be frequent. (Be aware, however, that these are also symptoms of other illnesses.)

- *Neglect of personal care hygiene and safety*, such as failure to bathe or wash, forgetting to undress before getting into bed, neglecting to launder clothing, ignoring traffic signals when out driving, or stepping out into traffic on busy roads.
- *Hallucinations, abnormal beliefs, anxiety and agitation:* some people become very anxious and exhibit mild paranoia before any other symptoms. A few forms of dementia manifest with hallucinations in the early stages. (Be aware, however, that these may also be symptoms of other conditions.)

It is important to remember that some conditions that are completely treatable may seem to mimic the symptoms of dementia. For example, someone who has a urinary tract infection (UTI) may become very confused and even aggressive. This infection is more common in older people and is treatable with antibiotics, after which the symptoms should subside. A UTI on its own is not a symptom of dementia.

A fall or blow to the head resulting in concussion may make someone confused and cause them to have problems with remembering what happened immediately before or after the injury. This is not a sign of dementia, but it does require medical attention as soon as possible.

Some medications can also cause people to be sleepy, confused or forgetful. If symptoms like this arise shortly after taking any new medication, consider first whether the medication is the cause. (This is a good time to state that you should always read the notes that come with a prescription drug, where all possible side effects are noted.)

Obviously, then, no one should assume that they have dementia or that someone they are close to has dementia unless all other possibilities have been excluded. Indeed, your doctor, if you consult them with worries about your cognition, should do certain blood and other tests and take a history – if possible, from someone close, to exclude other possibilities before referring you for a consultant opinion. If the doctor should diagnose dementia after a brief 'consulting room' test without referring you to a specialist, you should definitely question the diagnosis (although this is unlikely to happen). These comments also apply if you are a friend or relative who is concerned about a loved one and who is working with the doctor on their behalf. This means that if your loved one is diagnosed without the proper tests, ask for a referral to a specialist.

Worried about your memory?

A few years ago it was common to see this question on posters and flyers in libraries, doctors' surgeries and other information resources. We don't tend to see this question now, and there is a good reason for this. Generally, someone who has cognitive problems (memory issues) is not aware of this being so. We may consider that they are simply ignoring the issue – relatives commonly suggest that the person in question is 'in denial' – but if you forget things, you forget them: they are no longer in your 'memory', and even if someone reminds you about them ('I told you about that only this morning'), you do not recall this. You are more likely to think that the person who is reminding you is trying to trick you or catch you out. You know for certain that something did not happen or was not said *because you do not remember it*. It follows, then, that the person with memory problems is often not at all worried about their memory. So, in the list of symptoms above, we are usually considering those that someone else will notice.

Even if there are obvious problems with short-term memory, it does not follow that we are talking about dementia. Let us look closely at the 'symptoms' and differentiate between what happens to someone who is elderly and perhaps has MCI and someone who has the definite symptoms of dementia.

Check the symptoms
Memory loss

Any elderly (or not so elderly) person may complain about memory loss, but on questioning they would be able to provide examples of this, such as, 'I completely forgot where I had put my keys yesterday', or perhaps, 'I can never remember people's names'. In fact, difficulty in remembering names is a frequently reported worry in older people, most of whom do not have dementia.

Someone with dementia may not even realize that they have memory problems, may indeed vigorously deny this, and may accuse others of making things up when they are given examples of how they have forgotten something.

If you tell someone with dementia that they have asked you the same question several times, you are likely to get a look of incomprehension or even flat denial.

Many people with dementia can still remember the past very vividly and may give examples of these memories if you suggest they have a problem with their memory. A common example is someone who can recite from memory a long and complicated poem but cannot remember what you told them a few minutes before. One client was convinced that her husband had been misdiagnosed because 'He can still beat me at Scrabble every time we play.' As we will make clear later in this book, familiar skills such as reciting poems from memory, playing a familiar game or even driving can be retained for a long time after a diagnosis of dementia.

Disorientation

As we get older some of us may find we have to pause to recall directions clearly or may have to repeat directions to remember them or perhaps we need to write them down or use a map frequently, but we do not get lost in familiar places or forget the route home from the local shops, for example. People with dementia can and sometimes do get lost in familiar places and may on occasion be unable to retrace their route around a place they do not know well. For example, they may be unable to find their way back to the table after visiting the toilet when in a restaurant or another public place, or they may not return from a routine trip to the doctor or dentist because they have got lost. Sometimes people with dementia may even be disorientated within their own house, especially at night, if they have to get up to visit the toilet, for example.

Remembering

Older people can generally remember recent events, especially major events such as family celebrations, even if they do not recall all the conversations or people they met or the exact date of the event, but people with dementia may forget what happened yesterday, even if it was something important such as a grandchild's birthday party. They may, however, easily recall events in the far past with great clarity.

Everyday skills

Older people generally retain their social skills – things like shaking hands and saying 'thank you' and normal routines such as the sequence of events involved in washing or dressing themselves, even if it takes them longer to carry out these actions than when they were younger. Sometimes people with dementia can actually often retain outward social skills but lose interest in social activities or normal hobbies and pastimes, and may forget to wash or become unable to put on a simple article of clothing. Sometimes they may become unable to recognize an article of clothing or an everyday object. This kind of 'forgetting' may be occasional at first, but will become more common as the dementia progresses.

In our own homes most of us have familiar routines and
we can carry out tasks such as unloading the dishwasher
or putting out the rubbish without much thought.
Occasionally we may be distracted in the middle of carrying
out a task and leave it half done, but we will notice later
that we have done this. People with dementia often find
themselves unable to remember which cupboards to put
various items in; they may start a task and then become
distracted and leave it half done without recognizing this
(for example, they may leave a tap running and not notice);
or they may be unable to start a job like peeling vegetables
because they have forgotten what to do.

As people age they find it more difficult to learn new
skills or understand new appliances, and it may take several
attempts to learn how to manage the controls on (say) a
new dishwasher. However, unless they are simply being
perverse, they can, eventually, learn to use a new appliance.
People with dementia become unable to learn new things:
if a cooker is replaced, they may never learn to use the new
cooker, and most people with dementia become unable to
manage remote controls for the TV or other appliances.
Sometimes they can become confused and treat a remote
control as if it was a telephone or try to load dishes into the
washing machine.

Distraction

It can be harder to maintain attention as we get older –
we may be more easily distracted as we go about our daily
tasks, particularly as there are many more distractions

(radio, TV, internet, mobile phones) to divert us, but we are normally aware of this. If we find the washing-up not quite completed, for example, we will remember that the postman called and we were diverted from our task. Someone who has dementia will not manage to make this connection. If they find something out of place, they will not recall how this happened and are more likely to accuse others of being untidy or of 'hiding things'. Sometimes people with dementia become obsessed with 'putting things away' or 'making sure things are safe', and their family start to find things strangely out of place – handbags hidden under the bed, keys tucked away in unusual places, and so on. If this happens, the person responsible will not remember what they have done and may vigorously deny misplacing the bag or the key or even accuse others of deliberately hiding the item.

What can be done about MCI?

If MCI is not a disease and it is not dementia, why are we considering it at all? Why are you even reading this book?

The most recent research indicates that MCI affects many older people and, more importantly perhaps, that someone with MCI has a greater-than-average chance of being diagnosed with a form of dementia in the near future. It is, however, difficult to find the statistics to show the proportion of those with MCI who go on to develop dementia. This is partly because there are variations in what the experts consider qualifies as MCI (given that it is not a diagnosis in itself), and partly because there have not been many studies looking for the figures of progression.

One meta-analysis of 41 studies concluded that fewer than half of those with MCI would progress to dementia even after 10 years.[2] Other research suggests that 'Individuals with mild cognitive impairment (MCI) have a substantially increased risk of developing dementia due to Alzheimer's disease (AD)'.[3] Some doctors believe that roughly one-third of those with MCI are affected by medication or illness, and that they will make a recovery in due course.

It is known that MCI can be caused by many things – reaction to medication, serious infection, atmospheric pollutant, carbon monoxide poisoning, awakening suddenly from a deep sleep or even (some would argue) from a hangover because of over-indulgence in alcohol. But MCI caused by any of these things is a temporary condition. In due course we would expect the person affected to return to normal cognition in time. In this book we are generally concerned with MCI that has no obvious cause and that appears to be long term and gradually getting worse, or at least not improving.

What is generally believed and acknowledged is that people who have some cognitive impairment that stops short of a dementia diagnosis have a 'window of opportunity' to take steps to slow (or possibly even halt) any cognitive decline. This opportunity is not available after a diagnosis of dementia, and the reason for this is simple.

It is believed that actual dementia develops over a period of many (perhaps up to 20 or more) years.[4] If brain cells in a particular area of the brain die, they cannot regenerate. But the brain is a remarkable organ. When explaining dementia in my training sessions I often liken what happens to the experience of driving around a town. If a road is closed (perhaps due to road works), traffic will be diverted down a different route. Should you be taking this alternative route and find it congested because of, say, a traffic accident, you might turn off down a side road if you know the area and find your way to your destination by taking a series of diversions that do not constitute a direct route, but nevertheless get you where you plan to go.

When areas of the brain are damaged, the thinking, planning and actioning processes might need to take a longer route than the direct way, and the brain is very good at using such diversions to get to where it needs to go. Mostly we are unaware of this 'diversion' process. However, there is a limit. I always explain that symptoms of dementia appear when the brain has run out of 'alternative routes'. It can no longer find its way to the destination even using diversions. This is why people with dementia are unable to carry out the functions of everyday living. By this stage, any remedial action is no longer effective in restoring cognition, although Cognitive Stimulation Therapy (CST) and the various 'memory drugs' may slow decline (see pp.185–6).

Suppose that you have become aware of cognitive problems (or perhaps someone close to you has pointed them out) and you have consulted your doctor about this. They have run the relevant tests and perhaps you have been referred to a consultant who has given you a standard 'memory test' and even perhaps arranged for a scan of your brain. When the results of these tests are collated, your doctor tells you that there is no 'evidence' of dementia and that you simply have a 'mild cognitive impairment'.

Perhaps you will ask what you can do to help yourself in this situation. It is unlikely that you will be given any advice except the most broad general health advice, and you will simply be advised to return to see the doctor if you are worried in the future.

If this is your situation, this book is written for you.

Or consider that you have been worried about your cognition but have not consulted a doctor. Instead, you have looked things up (used the internet or a reference book) talked to your nearest and dearest and come to the conclusion that you do not have dementia; you are simply 'getting old' and slowing down. Now perhaps you are wondering if you can take any remedial steps to stop any further decline.

This book is written for people in your situation.

Whilst we do not know what causes dementia, we do know that there are a number of 'risk factors' that make it more likely. Because we do not know the ultimate cause of dementia, we also do not know whether addressing any of the known risk factors will prevent its onset, but it makes sense to try to address known risk factors and to make changes to our lifestyle that may help our cognition. We do know that some people 'recover' from MCI, and if we can improve our chances of such a recovery, why would we not attempt to do so?

There are a number of 'risk factors' for dementia, and these include low levels of education, certain social behaviours and lifestyle factors, cardiovascular disease, illnesses such as type 2 diabetes, certain head injuries and stroke, and poor nutrition, as well as some specific diseases that are rare. We can address some of these risk factors, but not all. For example, we cannot ensure that we will never suffer a head injury or heart attack, but we can take steps to improve our cardiovascular health and to guard against the development of maturity onset (type 2) diabetes.

In later chapters of this book we will be looking at some of the risk factors and learning how we can take steps to address them. Other chapters will consider memory aids that can help us to manage poor memory or cognitive problems, and factors that are thought to benefit cognition and keep us free from dementia.

Because some things in life are not certain, some chapters in this book will help you to look at practical steps you might take to plan for the future if your cognition gets worse and – just in case – what you can do if you eventually receive a diagnosis of dementia. There are also tips and advice for those helping someone with MCI or caring for someone in early stage dementia. There is a list of resources and organizations at the end of the book, in Chapter 10, for help and support.

In order to make this book as helpful as possible and to enable you to find the information you need to know without wading through information that may not be relevant to you at this time, there is a certain amount of repetition in various chapters. This means that if you begin by only wanting help and information about one area – memory aids, for example – you can go straight to that section of the book and find the information you need, together with pointers to other related aspects. You do not have to read through the entire book in order to find the advice you need.

If, on the other hand, you want to find out more about the general subject of cognition and MCI, then reading through the entire book will give you a good general background and you will be able to research in more depth with the help of the references that are given at the end of each chapter.

Above all, this is meant to be a 'self-help' book. Health professionals who are working with the elderly or anyone with MCI will find the book useful, but the ordinary reader who simply wants to help him or herself and to get information that is not easily available in the limited time given in a doctor's appointment should be able to find it easy to use.

I have tried to avoid technical 'jargon' or complicated medical terms and to keep the text clear, bearing in mind that if you have 'mild cognitive impairment', then the last thing you need is long explanations or complex sentences.

To clarify things further, each chapter includes a list of 'key points' so that you can find and focus on what you want and need to know.

Key points

- MCI is not a disease or a medical condition.
- MCI is not dementia and does not necessarily lead to dementia.
- There are many causes of MCI, and we do not know all of them.
- People with MCI can still function well enough to live independently.

- Many people with MCI are aware of their problems and want to help themselves.
- The advice in this book is meant to be both specific and practical.

Endnotes

1 See, for example, Jordan, M. (2014) *The Essential Carer's Guide to Dementia*. London: Hammersmith Health Books.

2 Mitchell, A.J. and Shiri-Feshki, M. (2009) 'Rate of progression of mild cognitive impairment to dementia – Meta-analysis of 41 robust inception cohort studies.' *Acta Psychiatrica Scandinavica*, 3 March. Available at https://doi.org/10.1111/j.1600-0447.2008.01326.x

3 Korolev, I.O., Symonds, L.L. and Bozoki, A.C. (2016) 'Predicting progression from Mild Cognitive Impairment to Alzheimer's Dementia using clinical, MRI, and plasma biomarkers via probabilistic pattern classification.' *PLoS One* 11, 2, e0138866.

4 Petersen, R.C. (2009) 'Early diagnosis of Alzheimer's disease: Is MCI too late?' *Current Alzheimer Research* 6, 4, 324–330.

Chapter 2

Practical Matters

Older people, whether they have mild cognitive impairment (MCI) or not, are wise to consider some practical steps to safeguard their financial position and their future welfare. We would all like to think that we will remain capable of managing our affairs until the end of our lives, that we will not be a 'burden' on our offspring or friends, that we will continue to enjoy the lifestyle we like and take part in activities we currently enjoy. Unfortunately for some of us this will not be the case. Becoming old and increasingly frail is a fact of life for most, and losing the ability to manage finances and take lifestyle decisions happens frequently enough that thinking ahead is wise.

Many people put off thinking about difficult matters such as frailty, cognitive decline and death because these are difficult and often depressing things to consider. But there is a positive side to taking action on these matters. By making a will, for example, you are ensuring that your beneficiaries inherit as you would wish; by making a power of attorney (POA), you are ensuring that your future financial, health and welfare matters will, if necessary, be managed by someone you trust; by considering your medical options, you can make your wishes clear for the future; and by tackling all these matters in good time, you can give yourself peace of mind about the future and feel able to enjoy the present without anxiety.

I have frequently heard people say that they will give attention to these matters 'when the time is right' or 'when I need to', but if you do become cognitively impaired and lose what is termed 'mental capacity', you will no longer be considered able to give POA to someone else, and it is possible that you will be considered to lack capacity to make a will. The law requires that anyone who makes a will or gives POA over their affairs to another must be cognitively able to understand what they are doing, so if you have MCI and have not made a will or considered who will manage your affairs if you are no longer able to do so, now is the time.

Who do you trust?

Drawing up a will, making a POA or considering health decisions are good moments to consider whom amongst your family, friends and relatives you are prepared to trust. Remember that when you give POA to someone, you are giving them the power to take decisions about your finances, your health and your welfare if you become unable to make these decisions yourself. Such a situation may not only arise in the case of dementia. If, for example, you have an accident or are taken ill and are unable to express your wishes, someone who has POA will be empowered to act on your behalf. If you are planning to make a lasting power of attorney (LPA), this is a good moment to have frank discussions with the family. You may believe that you all feel the same about something such as resuscitation or assisted suicide or residential care homes, but once you begin to talk about these subjects, you may be surprised. It is possible that a family member may carry out your wishes in any of these respects even if they do not agree with you, but it is also possible that they will not feel able to do so. It is important to discover someone's feelings in advance and whether they would feel able to act in the way you would choose.

Many people give POA to a child or children without thinking too hard about this because they assume that this is what they have to do or that this is the best thing to do. But the POA is given and not assumed – you choose who you would like to have it, although someone can refuse to accept a POA. Where someone who has not given POA becomes unable to manage their affairs, there is a legal process managed by the Court of Protection. The Court will appoint someone – called a 'deputy' – to manage the affairs of the person unable to manage their own. Usually this will be a family member or close friend, but the Court may appoint someone of their own choosing, such as a solicitor. So you can see that it is worthwhile giving careful consideration about who you would choose to make decisions on your behalf.

Extended family relationships

Families tend to be more complicated now than in the past, with divorce and second and subsequent marriages more common, and families more likely to include step relationships. One of the sad situations I have come across in my work is where people have forgotten to make changes to wills and POAs following changes in relationships. Many people are not aware that a subsequent marriage nullifies a previously made will, for example, and there are complications if an advance decision is made as well as an LPA (see below). Disagreements can arise within families as a result of past decisions about financial or welfare matters not being updated.

It is therefore important that you regularly review any financial and lifestyle decisions and the documents involved. Someone who has married again may wish to give POA to their new spouse, for example. An LPA can be changed or cancelled, but you have to remember to do this.[1]

Wills

Writing a will is something people often put off because it seems a morbid thing to do. People are also often under the impression that if they do not make a will everything will automatically go to their spouse or their children or their next of kin. However, this is not the case. If someone dies 'intestate', that is, without having made a will, there are strict criteria in law about how any estate they leave is distributed, and it may not be how the person would have chosen. This is especially true if someone has married again following bereavement or divorce or if someone is not married to their current partner.

For a will to be valid it must be made by someone who understands what they are doing. If someone develops dementia it does not mean that they lack capacity to make a will, but it might be harder for them to prove that they understand the implications of what they are doing.

If you have MCI and have not yet made a will, this is a good time to consider doing so. By making a will you can:

- Ensure that your wishes about any inheritance are made clear.
- Help your family in a time of distress to carry out your wishes.
- Simplify the administration of your estate after your death.

The action of writing a will might also help you to clarify your own feelings about relatives and any extended family, and help you to face the future with confidence.

A will does not have to be drawn up by a solicitor. It can be written on any plain sheet of paper or you can use a 'will form' that is obtainable at a stationers. There are even websites where you can use a template to write your will and download the finished document.[2] However, if your affairs are at all complicated, it is better to have the will document drawn up by an expert. Solicitors frequently have times of 'special offers' when the cost of drawing up a will is reduced or a reduced cost can be donated to charity, so do not be put off by thinking that you cannot afford it.

There has to be an 'executor' of a will, someone who will ensure that the instructions of the will are carried out. This can – but need not – be a solicitor or bank or anyone you care to name. It is quite common for husbands and wives to appoint each other as executor of their will and this can help to make life simpler, but if either partner has MCI or is at high risk of developing dementia, it might be more sensible to appoint someone else. It is worth remembering that if you appoint a bank or solicitor as executor, they will levy a fee, and this may make quite steep inroads into any inheritance you wish to leave to your family.

When your will has been made, signed and witnessed, make sure that you keep it in a safe place and that your family know where to find it. You do not have to lodge it with a solicitor or bank; indeed, they may charge a fee for keeping the will safe.

Power of attorney (POA)

Drawing up a POA means that someone (the 'donor') gives power to someone else (the 'attorney') to manage their affairs. In England there are two parts to an LPA: 'property and financial affairs' and 'health and welfare'. You can give POA for either one or for both. This means that you can choose to give someone else the power to manage your financial and property affairs and/or your health and welfare. You do not have to give POA for both, although a solicitor or other adviser may suggest that it is best that you do so.

Many people are reluctant to give POA to someone else because they fear that they will lose control over these areas of their life. It is important, however, to keep in mind that no one can see the future. It is possible that an accident or illness may make it impossible for you to handle these matters yourself, and should this happen, most people would like to think that a trusted person would manage things in the way that they would want them to be managed. Giving POA to someone you trust is one way to ensure that this happens.

You should choose someone you trust to have POA on your behalf, but it is important to make sure that you make your wishes known. If you have strong feelings about how your finances are managed or about what decisions are taken about your health and welfare, it is important that you take the time to talk to your attorney – and indeed, to your family in general – about your wishes. In my work I have frequently heard family members worrying about whether they are 'doing what Mum would have wanted' or 'making the right choice for Dad' because they have never had such discussions.

If you attempt to talk to your family about these important matters and they stop you and suggest you are 'being morbid' or 'worrying about nothing', be firm and press them to sit down and listen to your wishes. If you are unable to do this, you could write down your feelings and wishes and make sure that these notes are kept attached to the POA so that the attorney has some guidance if the occasion arises.

If you are worried about giving POA, it might reassure you to know that there are rules that your attorney must follow:

- They must follow any instructions and consider any preferences included in the LPA (you can write specific instructions about certain matters).

- They must also help you to make your own decisions as much as they can. This might involve giving simplified explanations or using pictures or asking you to indicate your feelings if you cannot speak.
- If they make any decisions, these must be in your best interests[3] and must respect your human and civil rights.

The procedures and rules about POA are complicated, and although you can draw up a POA yourself (you can download the form or send for forms to complete by post), many people prefer to get a solicitor to do the business for them.[4]

One thing to note: if you have perhaps thought well ahead and have already got an enduring power of attorney (EPA) in place, be aware that this is still perfectly valid (it will have been drawn up and signed before October 2007) and that you do not have to make a new LPA to cover your financial and property affairs. However, the EPA does not cover any health and welfare decisions.

An LPA needs to be registered with the Office of the Public Guardian before it is valid. An EPA is valid for use as soon as it is signed and witnessed, but if you become unable to manage your affairs (if, for example, you lose mental capacity), your attorney must register the EPA with the Office of the Public Guardian.

Property and finance
An LPA covering financial and property affairs means that your attorney can manage your money, pay your bills, run

your bank account, handle any investments and pension and benefit payments, and deal with matters of tax. It can be used as soon as it is registered, with your permission.

Health and welfare

An LPA for health and welfare covers decisions about medical treatment, where you are cared for and the type of care you receive, as well as day-to-day things like your diet, how you dress and your daily routine. It can only be used when you are unable to make your own decisions about these matters.

Advance statements and advance decisions

Some people have strong feelings about medical intervention and end-of-life care. An advance statement is a way of making your wishes clear to those who care for you and to medical staff. It covers preferences for both medical and personal lifestyle interventions, and can be referred to if you are no longer able (for whatever reason) to discuss what you would like to happen. Doctors and other medical health professionals may take your wishes into account if you have made an advance statement, but they are not legally bound to do so if they believe that your wishes are not in your best interests.

An advance decision is different as it sets out your wishes about refusing life-sustaining treatment in certain circumstances; it is legally binding in England and Wales.

Making an advance statement

Anyone can make an advance statement. It is sometimes called a 'living will' or a 'personal preference history'. Anyone who completes a 'This is me'[5] form to be referred to when going into hospital or residential care is effectively completing an advance statement. It can include wishes about domestic matters, finances, disclosure of information, care of domestic pets, nutritional matters or medical preferences. It is meant to make clear what your wishes and preferences are in case you are no longer able to explain these yourself. For example, you may be unconscious due to an illness or accident, you may be unable to speak following a stroke, or you may be confused and unable to be specific even though you are able to speak.

Someone who has an aversion to certain foods may wish to make this clear so that they are not presented with meals they feel unable to eat. Vegetarians or vegans may wish to state this in case they cannot choose their diets owing to one of the reasons stated above. If the welfare of a particular pet is very important to you and you have arrangements in place to care for them when you are no longer able to do so, you can make this clear in an advance statement. If a close friend or relative is aware of your wishes, you may want to state that this is the person who should be consulted on your behalf by health professionals about medical decisions. If you have a phobia or fear that would need to be taken into consideration when others are caring for you, an advance statement or living will is the place to make this clear.

An advance statement can be really helpful to those around you if you are not able, for whatever reason, to make decisions for yourself or to explain your needs and wishes. Remember, however, that it does not bind health professionals to a particular course of action and they may choose not to carry out your wishes about treatment if it conflicts with their professional judgement.

Making an advance decision

An advance decision may also be called an 'advance decision to refuse treatment' (ADRT), which indicates that it is a written statement of your wishes to refuse a particular treatment in a specific situation. If you make an ADRT, you are making sure that everyone knows what treatments you do not want to have if, in the future, you are unable to make your own decisions about this. It specifically allows you to state the conditions under which you will refuse life-sustaining treatment. For example, you may state that you do not wish to be fed or given fluids artificially if there is no reasonable hope of recovery.

An advance decision cannot be used to ask for something that is illegal – for example, euthanasia – and it cannot be used to refuse actions that are just meant to provide comfort, such as pain relief or warmth or hygienic measures. It is also worth noting that an advance decision does not allow you to say what particular treatment you would like – only what treatment you can refuse. It has to be worded very specifically and meet certain requirements that are set out in the Mental Capacity Act 2005.

If you just state your wishes verbally, this is an advance decision, but in certain situations the law says that it must be in writing. For example, an ADRT that refuses treatment to keep you alive (life-sustaining treatment), such as having your heart restarted (resuscitation) or being put on a breathing machine (ventilator), must be:

- written down
- signed by you (or if you are unable to sign you can ask someone who is with you to sign)
- witnessed.

It must say exactly what treatment you want to refuse and in which situation. This is because you may want to refuse a treatment in a particular situation but not in another. It must also contain a statement such as, 'I refuse this treatment, even if my life is at risk as a result', to make it legal.

One thing to note: if you make an ADRT and then later give POA to someone that includes the authority to accept or refuse treatment on your behalf, the ADRT becomes invalid. If you have strong feelings about refusing life-saving treatment, you should be aware of this and make sure that your attorney is too.

Moving house

This subject is covered in more detail in Chapter 7. One situation I have often come across in my work is where younger family members consider that someone they care for should move house or move to residential care because they are finding it difficult to give support when required. One son told his mother, 'You will have to move because

I live too far away. If you have a problem it is difficult for me to get over to help.' Consider how this made his mother feel. There was no discussion about any alternative support measures that might be put in place. She told me that she felt her son's only concern was his own convenience, that the physical upheaval of moving plus the loss of all of her well-known support networks was of no interest to him.

Driving

There are rules about possession of a driving licence.[6] Someone who has MCI is not compelled to tell the DVLA (Driver and Vehicle Licensing Agency) about this, but you should consider carefully whether you feel competent to continue driving. Most of us would feel that we would lose a lot of the feeling of independence if we could no longer drive, although there are other things to consider:

- Do you feel confident when you are driving? Many people are very nervous drivers and would actually rather not drive, especially on routes that are not familiar. If you do not feel confident when driving, then being able to drive is not really increasing your independence.
- Are you certain that your eyesight is sufficient to make you a safe driver? If your optometrist has suggested that you should not drive, you should take notice of this.
- Do you have other physical conditions that limit your ability to move about? For instance, can you turn

your head easily to look over your shoulder if you are reversing?

- Are you confident about finding your way around? More and more people rely on a 'sat nav' to help them with route finding, and whilst these are very useful devices, you should still feel able to find your way by reading route signs if necessary. Simple things like roadworks and diversions can mean that the sat nav-recommended route may not always work, and sat navs will not tell you about narrow roads or difficult routes you should avoid.

Giving up your driving licence may seem unthinkable at first, but there are many alternatives to driving yourself around. For instance, there may be another family member who would be willing to do the driving when you go out. In towns public transport is usually very good and for seniors bus travel is free outside of busy times. Train travel, too, can be highly convenient, and seniors can obtain cheaper travel 'railcards'.

There is more discussion about driving and alternatives in Chapter 4 of this book.

Thinking about care homes and other options

The remarks I have made above also apply to the sticky subject of care homes and residential care. Most of us hope that the situation when we need to be 'put into a home' will never arise. In my work I have come across many people who have made their relatives promise that they will never 'put them in a home', and I have had to support many family members who needed to face the decision to pursue the residential care option with great reluctance. I generally advise families to be careful about any promises they may make. There are times when a residential care home or nursing home is the only or best option, and it can be hard to live with the guilt of a broken promise.

Rather than force your family to make a promise they may not be able to keep, why not take steps to ensure that your wishes can be accommodated? First, you can make financial plans for your care options. You may not meet the criteria for state financial assistance for care home fees and you may have to consider a financial plan to take this into account. Such plans are complex and you would be wise to seek the advice of a specialist for this. The cost of specialist advice may be worth it if you obtain peace of mind in this matter. You may also be able to so organize your finances that you can pay for 'live-in' care and need never contemplate communal residential care.

Second, rather than refusing to even consider the possibility of residential care you might think about deciding instead what is important to you about your own lifestyle and what would make you happier to accept this option. For example, you might discuss what support your family are able to give you or would be able to give you in the future. Bear in mind that you and your family may have different views on your ability to cope with life's vagaries. Your family – particularly your children – will be seeing things from a younger, more vigorous point of view, and may consider that (for example) using cook/chill ready meals instead of cooking from scratch is a poor choice. If you become unable to cook a main meal, however, you may decide that a thawed and reheated ready meal is acceptable. Younger family carers may think that your housekeeping habits are poor and that you are no longer able to maintain your house properly. It may be that you consider their standards to be unacceptably high, but it is better to talk something like this through and perhaps consider employing a cleaner once a week rather than face endless criticism about something you feel is not important. Your children may feel that you can no longer manage your shopping adequately, although you think that with a little help – perhaps a lift to the shops and some help with heavy carrying – you could continue to be independent. In such a case maybe you could ask someone to set up a monthly online order to be delivered to the house, which would include heavy articles, so that a short walk to the shops every couple of days would mean that you could continue to manage the rest. Small measures like this, if arranged carefully and accepted gracefully, can make the difference between 'managing' and 'needing' to go into a home.

Third, why not face up to the possibility – however remote – that you may need residential care at some time in the future? Think carefully about your likes and dislikes in this regard. By doing this you can continue to be in control of your lifestyle.

One common misconception people have is that the residential care home is like a prison. Indeed, I came across this myself in my work when one daughter of a client said that she could not possibly consider a care home for her mother as her mother enjoyed going out so much. When I followed up, it turned out that she had thought that, as she put it, 'Once they have gone into the home they are not allowed out.' I was able to reassure her that she could continue to take her mother out as often as she wished. Except in certain circumstances,[7] a residential care home is supposed to be 'a home' for the residents and not a place in which they are confined.

People will often quote 'loss of independence' as an objection to moving into a care home, and it is interesting to discuss what this phrase actually means. Is it, for example, the wish to rise and to go to bed at a time of your choosing, to eat the meals you desire and when you feel hungry, to walk to the shops when you choose or to go out into the garden as desired to join an activity when you want to or to avoid activity if you wish?

Or are your objections to do with a dislike of communal living as such? Perhaps you are a very private person and would dislike sharing communal areas or eating or watching TV with others. Perhaps your objections are to do with the suggestion that others would be involved in your intimate personal care, even if you are able to manage this yourself?

Whatever your objections to the suggestion of a residential care home, thinking them through, expressing them to your family and making clear what is important to you can only be a positive step. If you decide that your main objection to residential care is (say) having to share a bathroom with others, you at least know that the most important criteria for you is an en suite facility in your room. If your family know that having a cooked breakfast and being able to step out into the garden whenever you wish (these are my own preferences) are of vital importance to you, then at least they know what to look for if they are choosing a home on your behalf.

Think about what you want in different situations, discuss things with your family or attorney, and above all, *write them down*. In this way you will feel able to remain in control of your life and, if the worst happens and others have to act for you, they will know what your wishes are.

Why think about these things?

You may wonder why I have included information about these difficult areas in a book about helping yourself when you have MCI. The truth is that in my work with people who have MCI, people who have a diagnosis of dementia, and their families and carers, I have frequently had to support those who have found it very difficult to make decisions on another's behalf and others who have had to struggle with the slow processes of the law when no prior arrangements have been made and their loved one becomes unable to manage legal and welfare matters themselves.

We would all like to think that families will 'pull together' or maintain the welfare of the person they are caring for as their main criteria when they are having to make financial and welfare decisions. But different family members can have different views on what is 'the best thing' for the person they care for. If families and carers are also having to cope with different advice from various health professionals and legal advisers, it can make life complicated and caring very onerous. By stating your wishes clearly and writing them down you will not only reduce the burden on those caring for you, but also ensure that your wishes will be acted on.

Key points

- Consider practical matters, especially legal matters, in good time. Do not wait for an 'emergency'.
- Everyone should make a will. It does not have to be expensive or complicated.
- Giving POA to someone you trust is a sensible precaution.
- You can only give POA to another person if you have mental capacity, so it is better not to delay doing this.
- Think carefully about who you trust best to carry out your wishes if you are unable to manage financial things yourself.
- Write down your wishes about future healthcare and medical interventions so that others know what you would like.
- It is a good idea to discuss your wishes with your family in advance.
- Consider matters that might arise such as having to give up driving, needing to move house or needing nursing home care, and let your family know your wishes about these matters. This is empowering both for you and for them.

Endnotes

1 Instructions about how to change or cancel an LPA are available at www.gov.uk/power-of-attorney

2 See, for example, www.gov.uk/make-will

3 See www.gov.uk/make-decisions-for-someone/making-decisions

4 Information and forms can be downloaded from www.gov.uk/power-of-attorney

5 www.alzheimers.org.uk/get-support/publications-factsheets/this-is-me

6 See www.gov.uk/driving-medical-conditions

7 See the Deprivation of Liberty safeguards, outlined in the Mental Capacity Act 2005.

Chapter 3

Physical Health

Our physical health has a direct bearing on our cognition. Anyone who has had days when they feel 'under the weather' and decided that they cannot tackle tasks that need extra concentration will understand this. Some physical conditions such as urinary tract infections (UTIs) are known and acknowledged to be a common cause of confusion in elderly people, even those without a diagnosis. However, recent research indicates that dementia may itself be caused by infections.[1] We just do not yet know all the facts around this set of diseases.

It can sometimes be difficult to understand that most of the dementias are actually physical diseases, not mental disease. This confusion can arise because in the early stages of dementia no physical symptoms are usually apparent. People often seem physically very healthy. Clients have stated to me things like, 'My mother is physically very well – she is never ill. It is just her memory which is causing concern.' The very fact that the diagnosis is often made by a psychiatrist can confuse patients even further.

In Alzheimer's disease and other dementias, physical changes take place in the tissues of the brain and these changes can be seen on a brain scan – this is why a brain scan is now commonly ordered before a diagnosis is made. Only a few years ago the diagnosis of 'probable dementia' was frequently made on the basis of observation, questioning of close informants (such as immediate family) and 'memory tests'.

A brain scan will show signs such as widespread cerebral atrophy (wasting away) particularly affecting the parts of the brain known as the parietal and temporal lobe regions. These physical changes affect the way the brain works, making memory and other cognitive processes more difficult. If any other visible part of the body – for example, the hand – was to 'waste away' in the same way, most people would rapidly understand that it would be impossible for the person affected to use the hand normally. However, we cannot see the brain and there is a temptation to feel that the person whose brain is affected is just 'not trying hard enough' or that they are 'allowing themselves' to be overcome by apathy.

So the first important thing is to recognize that dementia is a physical disease that causes deterioration in brain tissue.

It is sensible, then, to takes steps to optimize physical health if there is any indication of mild cognitive impairment (MCI). This is not to suggest that you should become health obsessed, but it makes sense to take better care of your health as you grow older. Older people have a less robust immune system, and even simple infections and minor illness can involve a longer recovery time. You may have already noticed this yourself – perhaps you take longer to get over a cold or a minor injury. Because we are used to modern medicine producing treatment for many of the severe diseases that were untreatable in the past (and even producing cures for some of them), there is a tendency to think that illness doesn't really matter and that it has only a short and limited effect on the body: after suitable 'treatment' we will be cured and not troubled with the symptoms of this illness again.

Unfortunately, this is frequently not the case, and it is important to recognize and understand this. For example, operation scars can be painful, itchy or unsightly, and keloid scar tissue might form or numbness may be a problem. Childhood illness like polio may result in 'post polio syndrome'; chicken pox may resurface as shingles; gastric illness may have a long-term effect on the digestive system; a simple cold may result in long-term sinusitis or trigger an asthma attack; rheumatic fever can result in heart problems – the list is seemingly endless. As already pointed out, it is known that any physical illness or infection is likely to result in a drop in cognitive abilities in someone who has a diagnosis of dementia, so it is clear that physical illness does have an effect on our brain.

How, then, can we best look after our physical health in older life?

Nutrition

We often see the slogan 'You are what you eat', and it is indeed true that our nutritional status can make a difference to our general health. Epidemiology studies from the past indicate that one of the prime reasons for a general improvement in the health of a population is not due to medical advances but to an improvement in general nutritional status. For example, just a small reduction in levels of certain vitamins can result in deficiency diseases. The human body only needs quite a small amount of vitamin C to prevent scurvy (a deficiency disease), but the lack of that small amount caused severe illness and death amongst sailors – whose diet was usually ship's biscuits and salted meat – before this knowledge became known. Vitamin C is found in fresh foods, particularly fresh fruit and vegetables.

Nutrition is one of the most discussed subjects in connection with diseases that have an (at present) unknown 'cause'. Diseases such as arthritis, Alzheimer's, irritable bowel syndrome, some forms of Parkinson's disease, multiple sclerosis and fibromyalgia are all hypothesized as having a nutritional cause and/or cure.

It is difficult sometimes to understand what the best diet is for a healthy life as we are bombarded with slogans that suggest we should 'eat five a day', 'cut visible fat from meat', 'go gluten free', 'reduce meat consumption', 'eat a good varied diet', 'avoid strong sunlight' and above all, 'trust our doctor's advice'.

Some of the most common advice regarding 'healthy eating' does not bear up to close investigation. For example, the suggestion that we should keep to a low-fat diet is so prevalent that it is commonly accepted as truth. It may be that this is sound advice for someone in mid-life hoping to avoid heart disease (although there is no actual robust evidence to bear this out), but for someone in later life hoping to avoid dementia, this may be the very worst advice of all. Fats provide energy for the growth and maintenance of body tissues and the fat-soluble vitamins A, D and E are all found in edible fats. To supply the fatty acids necessary for the proper functioning of the brain we need to consume at least 15 grams of fat each day. Fat is particularly important to the brain – we need a steady intake of fat for the brain to function properly.[2]

Cholesterol, too, is a fatty substance (known as a 'lipid') and is vital for the normal functioning of the body. Cholesterol is needed everywhere in the brain to manufacture neurotransmitters, the means by which nerves communicate. To the general public, however, cholesterol is a real 'baddie' to be avoided at all costs. This belief is the result of years of persuasive publicity and misinformation based on what is now known to be a faulty piece of research. It may even be that low blood cholesterol is one of the factors that makes us susceptible to developing dementia.[3]

What exactly is a 'good varied diet'? And what should we do when one set of advice contradicts another? When considering diet recommendations, especially those published in the popular press, it is worth going back to the source and assessing the credibility or otherwise of the initial recommendation. Diet advice can spread quickly and easily becomes distorted as it is spread, so that a simple advertising slogan or suggestion from a celebrity in the media can be taken up and repeated until it comes to be believed as a fact.

So, rather than considering what diet recommendations we *should* follow, it might be worth looking instead at some of the accepted 'facts' and deciding if they are worthy of attention:

- *'Facts' like: Salad is a particularly healthy food.* In fact, salad items are simply vegetables (and sometimes fruits) that can be eaten raw. A plate of salad is no healthier than a plate of cooked vegetables. Salad is fine to eat if you like it and it is low in calories, but it is possible to eat a healthy diet and never eat a plate of salad.
- *'Facts' like: Potatoes are bad for you and have less food value than other vegetables.* Potatoes are a starchy vegetable, and if you are trying to lose weight, you may like to restrict the amount you eat, but they are not intrinsically bad for you. White potatoes are actually lower in calories than sweet potatoes; they are a source of fibre in our diet and also a source of vitamin C, especially if you leave the skin on.
- *'Facts' like: Eggs are high in cholesterol and should not be eaten every day.* Eggs are a very important food source, rich in protein and vitamins B2, B12 and D, as well as many trace elements important for the body to function. It is now known that the cholesterol in food has very little effect on blood cholesterol levels.
- *'Facts' like: Eating fruit is important for our health.* Fruits are generally high in vitamin C and also provide fibre in our diet. However, vegetables are also high in vitamin C and a source of fibre. Generally, you can

consider fruit and vegetables to be interchangeable as far as food value is concerned. If you don't like vegetables, eat more fruit; if you don't like fruit, eat more vegetables.

- *'Facts' like: Vegetarians are healthier than meat-eaters.* A vegetarian diet or a vegan diet can be healthy (although vegans have to take care to balance the types of food they eat), and some people claim to lose weight on a vegetarian diet, but a diet that includes meat and/or fish can be just as healthy. Reducing the calorific value of what you eat will result in weight loss, whether you include meat and fish in the diet or not.

The recommendation to eat a 'varied diet' is sound advice because in this way you will have an intake of all the nutrients necessary for your health and will not be excluding any important food groups. So, the best advice might be to have as unrestricted a diet as possible and to enjoy experimenting with different foods and new ways of cooking so that you always look forward to your meals and enjoy eating without the temptation to overeat.

The lesson from this is that so-called food 'facts' are not all that they may seem. Try not to be led astray by the things you read in the media, even if they appear to be backed by medical advice. The body has a way of extracting the nutrients it needs from what you eat, and your diet would have to be strange and restricted indeed to have a marked impact on your health.

Choosing your healthcare advisers

> If the doctor tells me to take a pill, I take it. I don't ask about it – that's his business.

> I was seeing the doctor for a routine health check and she asked me my age. When I said 66 she said 'But you're not on any medication. That's ridiculous at your age!'

It is not always safe to make the assumption that 'a qualified doctor knows what's best' (Irwig *et al.* 2014, p.53)[4] for our health as it is so difficult for any health professional to keep up to date with the latest research into treatments and tests. This is not to suggest that you should ignore your doctor's advice or omit to seek help when you have a health problem. But you should use your doctor intelligently. The days of the doctor who knew you from birth and understood your family background are long gone. Your doctor should be employed as you would with any other professional. A financial adviser might suggest some investment but they would expect you to make the decision about whether to go ahead. A solicitor might have a greater knowledge of the law but they always act under your instructions. Consider the doctor (or any other health professional) in the same light. They may have a greater knowledge and experience of the health matter you are consulting about, but no one knows your own body better than you.

 In their very sensible book, *Smart Health Choices*, Professor Les Irwig, Judy Irwig, Dr Lyndal Trevena and Melissa Sweet suggest that you can judge a health practitioner's decision-making skills by whether they are using the best evidence available and are prepared to share this information with you whilst at the same time taking account of your preferences.[5] It may be difficult to know whether your adviser is using the best evidence available (or any evidence at all), but you yourself can look up evidence for health decisions.

Some doctors are better at sharing information than others and some patients really do not want too much information – it is up to you to decide – but if you do want information about your condition or your treatment, then view with suspicion any health practitioner who is reluctant to give you as much information as you want. I would also suggest you be wary of someone who speaks in jargon or uses language that you find difficult to understand. Why use the term 'aphasia' instead of 'difficulty with speaking' unless you are talking to someone you know understands the term? It is true that a doctor is learned in medical terminology, but when patients are consulting them, a good doctor should be able to express him or herself in plain language.

When it comes to treatment for any medical condition there is always a choice – even if that choice is to refuse all medical intervention. If your health practitioner forgets to ask you about your own preferences or to discuss options with you, you might consider changing to another adviser. It is very simple to change an NHS doctor in the UK and you do not have to give a reason for doing so. If, on the other hand, you are paying for care or treatment as a private patient, you can simply terminate your agreement with the practitioner concerned. If your doctor refers you to a specialist consultant, you do not have to accept that referral. Indeed, it is now more common for the doctor to ask the patient to choose their own consultant from an online database.

In the UK it is common for older people to think that they have to accept whatever the doctor advises and to be referred to wherever the doctor decides, but this is not the case. If you are getting treatment via the NHS it does not mean that you are not paying for it. Whilst the NHS is 'free at the point of delivery', it is not free, it is not charity, and you are entitled to have your own preferences considered.

If you have MCI, it is important to take charge of your own health, and this may mean refusing medication if you do not agree with the prescription; pressing for a particular drug to be prescribed if this is appropriate; or asking for a referral to a specialist even if your doctor does not think it necessary. The most important thing, however, is to make sure that your main healthcare adviser (and this will most often be your doctor) understands your health and your concerns, keeps up to date with the latest research (or at least listens if you draw their attention to the latest research), consults your preferences and answers your questions.

Surgery

When I opted for a breast reconstruction following my breast cancer, I did not realize that it would involve several operations.

I thought a hip replacement was a routine procedure but I suffered a stroke afterwards and my life has not been the same since.

No one explained that a simple cataract operation could go wrong. Now I am blind in one eye.

Surgery is another area of health we tend to take for granted these days. Many surgical operations are classified as 'minor procedures', which can lead us to believe that there are no risks attached to them and that recovery will be quick and uneventful. When I question clients about their past medical history, I am often taken aback by a long list of surgical interventions that have led up to the present breakdown in health. It is one thing to acknowledge that with modern surgical knowledge and expertise people can now be cured of problems that would have left them disabled for life in the past, and quite another to casually undergo surgery and the risks of a general anaesthetic without giving consideration to the risks that are always attached.

Doctors are bound to detail the risks to patients and are careful to do so, but as a relative once said to me, 'When he said that 10 per cent of patients are left with a limp, I assumed I would be one of the other 90 per cent.' So, be sure that you have understood any risks and thought about the possibility that you may be 'one of the 10 per cent'.

Surgical procedures are sometimes necessary as a matter of life and death and are sometimes important to ensure a good quality of life; in these cases most people would be prepared to accept the risk of post-operative infection or of an adverse reaction to a general anaesthetic, but it is nevertheless important if you have MCI to consider carefully before undergoing any surgical procedure. It is very likely that any minor cognitive problems will become worse in the initial period after the procedure, and in some cases, cognition does not recover completely.

If a surgical procedure (even a minor one) is necessary, consider a preparation beforehand often known as 'prehab' (pre-habilitation), in which patients are guided on how to prepare for an operation and hospital stay by being encouraged to boost their general fitness and mental well-being before a procedure. This is a relatively new concept, but the Royal College of Anaesthetists (whose initiative this is) suggests that patients taking part in prehab schemes have a 50 per cent reduction in complications such as pneumonia, and that their hospital stay is cut by up to three days.[6]

Minor health matters and infections

Without becoming health obsessed, don't neglect minor health matters. Maybe you struggled into work with a bad cold in the past or ignored small injuries or 'worked through' a mild virus infection. Many of us did the same as young fit individuals and felt none the worse for it. But as you grow older, your recovery time is likely to be longer, and neglecting minor matters may cause them to become more serious. If you get a cold or a minor infection you should treat it sensibly, rest more and take your doctor's advice. If you have any chronic health condition such as diabetes you should take extra care, even during a mild illness. Diabetes is considered to be a high-risk factor for later development of dementia, and you should always treat it seriously.

Most people reading this book are likely to have retired from full-time employment, so make the most of your ability to take life more slowly and rest when it is important to do so.

Exercise

I don't want to join a gym at my age.

More than any other lifestyle factor (apart from giving up smoking), taking regular exercise is considered to be beneficial for general physical health and mental health. Physical exercise improves cardiovascular health and lowers the risk of coronary heart disease and stroke, and it is also considered to lower the risk of some cancers, of osteoarthritis and depression. These may seem to be somewhat nebulous claims, but perhaps more interesting for any older person is that regular exercise reduces the risk of falls.

If you have not experienced a fall since you were a child, you may wonder why this fact is significant, but if you have had a fall in the past year or so, you will understand. Apart from any injury sustained, a fall causes a huge loss of confidence in an older person. Even just one fall can mean that you become more fearful of negotiating steps, rough ground or difficult paths. Each time you avoid a potential obstacle 'in case you might fall' it compounds the loss of confidence. A severe fall can even be the cause of 'flashbacks' where you relive the fall all over again. You may begin to walk more slowly, to avoid certain routes, and to go out less or to only go out if you are accompanied.

In addition to the effect on feelings of confidence, injuries – even minor injuries that are sustained as a result of a fall – can have lasting results. As we age it takes longer to get over small hurts. If you are on blood-thinning medications, even small injuries can cause bruising and bleeding. If you are diabetic, a small injury may have serious repercussions. A neglected minor injury can lead to complications and further medical intervention.

Regular exercise, then, is an important thing to include in your lifestyle. Some people dislike the very thought of exercise because to them it brings back memories of school PE lessons or they associate the word with gyms full of sweating people wearing Lycra, or because the word 'exercise' suggests running and weight lifting, and such activities bore them. However, many things constitute exercise; playing tennis, bowling, swimming, gardening, walking and carrying bags of shopping are all forms of exercise.

You do not have to join a club or a gym in order to increase your level of physical activity. Think creatively about this. You could join a local 'Walking for Health' group or you could simply decide to walk for 20 minutes around the neighbourhood on several days a week. You could sign up for an exercise class at your local leisure centre if you wanted to, but you could just as well use an exercise video at home a few times a week. You could rent an allotment or just decide to do more of the gardening yourself instead of leaving it to your partner or a gardener. You could join a cycling club or you could just cycle or walk to the shops instead of always taking the car.

Even if you have mobility problems it is likely that there is some form of exercise you could incorporate into your lifestyle. If you can't run, you can walk; if you can only walk slowly, you can decide to walk more; if you can't stand for very long, you can do a chair exercise class; if you need to spend many hours sitting down, you can move your feet and your hands and change your position regularly. Whatever exercise you are able to do is likely to be of benefit. Of course you should take your doctor's advice if necessary (for example, if you have a chronic condition that inhibits exercise), but keeping the body mobile is important for your physical health, and interestingly, it is now also considered to be important for your continuing mental health. There is more information on this in Chapter 5.

Eyesight

Few people escape some eyesight problems as they age. Almost every older person suffers from presbyopia or an inability to focus clearly on near objects. Reading glasses can help with this problem. However, other eye problems such as cataracts, glaucoma and macular degeneration are all more common as we age. Some of these conditions can be helped by medication and some claims are made that certain foods help eye health. One important thing to remember is the big part that the brain plays in vision. Put simply, our eyes take in the light but it is our brain that interprets what we see. Surgical solutions to problems like cataracts make adjustments to the eye, but in every case it is necessary following the operation for the brain to 'relearn' what it is interpreting. Long-term wearers of spectacles will be familiar with being told that they need to 'get used to' a new lens prescription, so will understand this more easily.

For this reason it is worth ensuring that cataract surgery is carried out whilst the brain can still adapt itself easily. If you have MCI, this could be a good time to look at eye health and to ensure any corrections necessary are carried out as soon as possible.

If your eyesight is very poor and you are going to be given any memory tests by your doctor or a specialist, make sure that they know this. The test involves some visual work, and large-print versions of the test can be made available if you let the clinic know in advance.

An inability to see clearly can affect many of our everyday activities, so it is important to get the best eye healthcare that you can. Some optometrists specialize in eye health in elderly people, and it may be worth using such a specialist instead of a general optician in order to make sure that you get some specialized advice. If you are diabetic, it is particularly important to pay attention to your eye health and not neglect regular check-ups and vision checks.

Hearing

Hearing loss is extremely socially isolating, and it is now known that age-related hearing loss has a small but significant association with cognitive decline and dementia. Studies suggest that a hearing impediment is associated with a 30–40 per cent rate of accelerated cognitive decline.[7] The reasons are still not completely clear, but one suggestion is that when there is a loss of hearing, greater cognitive resources are required for auditory perception, and that this diverts resources away from processes such as working memory.[8] Put simply, your brain is diverting resources away from 'thinking' in order to listen better. Since some hearing loss is common in everyone as they age, this suggestion is very significant.

It is not yet clear whether correcting hearing loss by use of hearing aids alters the risk for dementia. However, even the limited information and knowledge we have should suggest that it is important to take care to protect your hearing. When using noisy machines and tools, always use ear defenders. Music should not be played louder than is necessary, and this area of research should make us question the over-use of ear buds and other in-ear devices. There is no cure for age-related hearing loss.

If we consider the supposition that for those hard of hearing the effort to hear diverts resources away from other cognitive functions, we might also take other precautions. Do not strain to hear if you can improve the situation by moving to a quieter place, turning up the volume, closing down distracting background sound or using other senses (sight, touch) to help in understanding what is being said. Keep away from noisy environments. If it has been suggested that you need a hearing aid, invest in the best you can afford and take the trouble to get used to it so that it becomes an 'aid' and not a distraction.

We should not ignore the isolation that comes from being unable to hear others and the fact that this can isolate people with hearing loss irrespective of any theories about cognition. If you find it difficult to hear a conversation, the tendency is to withdraw from the conversation and human contact, and perhaps to find consolation in solitary pursuits that do not involve others. It is known that continued social contact reduces the risk of developing dementia, and so anything that discourages both this and networking must be a bad thing.[9]

This fact, again, should encourage us all to take charge of our environment in order to maximize the ability to hear what is going on around us, to take steps to avoid any further damage to our hearing, and to make use of any aids that enable us to hear and to take part in human social intercourse. For example, you could make use of hearing aids, hearing loops, lip reading, subtitles or simply turning down the volume on background noise such as the radio and TV. There are now phone 'apps' that translate spoken words into written words to help those who are hearing impaired to follow conversations.[10] More information can be found about this in Chapter 10.

Associated illness

Certain physical illnesses have an association with dementia, or in some cases, raise its risk factor. If you have an illness where the risk of dementia is very high, your medical adviser will have made you aware of this fact and you will also be given specific advice. But there are some chronic conditions that may predispose you to cognitive problems, and if you are aware of this you can take steps to mitigate against developing problems:

- Heart disease may predispose you to vascular dementia. Do not ignore existing heart disease; take proper medical advice and follow your doctor's recommendations. Vascular dementia is one of the dementias that can be dramatically helped by addressing the heart condition that predisposes towards it.

- Stroke may be recovered from, but in some cases it may result in dementia. Recovery from stroke, more than any other disease, is often improved by the effort of the patient themselves. It is also not widely known that recovery from stroke can continue for many years after the stroke itself, so do not believe anyone who suggests that you should now 'accept your limitations' and give up any rehabilitation attempts. Further information about stroke recovery is given in Chapter 10.

- Diabetes is a high risk factor for dementia. It is a serious disease and should not be treated lightly.

The number of people diagnosed with diabetes is rising, but latest research shows that you can possibly achieve remission of your diabetes with proper attention to health and diet.[11] Because this disease can now be treated (but not cured) with medication, the temptation is to accept the diagnosis as just 'bad luck' and to take the medicine assuming that you will have the condition for life and that if things get worse you can always increase the medication to compensate. But diabetes is not an inevitable result of ageing; it is a disease that you can actively do something to address. It also has serious consequences in terms of general health – eyesight, circulation and cognition can all be affected as a side effect of diabetes. It is a disabling disease and should be treated seriously.

- If you carry a particular gene that already raises your risk of dementia then herpes simplex virus and some other viruses may increase your risk of dementia even more. It is not likely that you will know whether you carry a particular gene, but as stated above, we can all take greater care of our general health and treat minor infections with care.

- People who experience anaesthetic delirium after an operation are at higher risk of developing dementia. If you have experienced this, avoid unnecessary minor surgery and always ensure that your surgeon knows that you have experienced this previously. Some quite major surgical interventions can now be carried out without a general anaesthetic thanks to advances in techniques.

If you have any of these associated conditions and are also considered to have MCI, take extra care to maintain optimum health and follow the advice of your healthcare adviser.

This chapter has discussed the way that physical health and minor ailments may have an effect on your cognition. We know that dementia is a physical illness and that it is associated with other physical ailments. No one wishes to allow worries about their physical health to preoccupy them to the exclusion of being able to enjoy later life, but some careful thought and sensible lifestyle measures can give you the best chance of ensuring that any MCI does not develop into a diagnosis of dementia.

Key points

- Dementia is a physical condition and not a mental health problem.
- If you have MCI, this is a good time to reassess your lifestyle.
- Optimize your nutritional status.
- Check that you still need all prescription medication and that it is not interfering with your cognition (thinking and memory).
- Consider exercising more.
- Pay attention to eyesight and hearing problems.
- Make sure you attend to any long-term medical problems.

Endnotes

1   Kumar, D., Kumar, V., Choi, S.H., Kevin, J., *et al.* (2016) 'Amyloid-peptide protects against microbial infection in mouse and worm models of Alzheimer's disease.' *Science Translational Medicine 8*, 340, doi:10.1126/scitranslmed.aaf1059

2   Haag, M. (2003) 'Essential fatty acids and the brain.' *Canadian Journal of Psychiatry*. Available at https://doi.org/10.1177/070674370304800308

3   Lorin, H. (2006) *Alzheimer's Solved (Condensed Edition)*. CreateSpace Independent Publishing Platform.

4   Irwig, L., Irwig, J., Trevena, L. and Sweet, M. (2014) *Smart Health Choices: Making Sense of Health Advice*. London: Hammersmith Health Books.

5   Ibid, p.79.

6   See www.rcoa.ac.uk

7   Lin, F.R., Ferrucci, L., An, Y., Goh, J.O., *et al.* (2013) 'Association of hearing impairment with brain volume changes in older adults.' *Neuroimage 90*, 84–92.

8   Lin, F.R. and Albert, M. (2014) 'Hearing loss and dementia – Who is listening?' *Aging & Mental Health 18*, 6, 671–673. doi:10.1080/13607863.2014.915924

9   University College London (2019) 'Socially active 60-year-olds face lower dementia risk.' *ScienceDaily*, 2 August. Available at www.sciencedaily.com/releases/2019/08/190802144414.htm

10 See, for example, Live Transcribe, an Android app: www.android.com/accessibility/live-transcribe

11 www.diabetes.org.uk/research/research-round-up/research-spotlight/research-spotlight-low-calorie-liquid-diet

Chapter 4

Lifestyle – Activities of Daily Living (ADLs)

What on earth are activities of daily living (ADLs)?

You have probably never come across this term, but health professionals involved with dementia care use it all the time. So what are 'activities of daily living' (or ADLs)? Generally, this term is used to include the things we do every day – or at least on a regular basis – to carry out our daily lives. Think washing, dressing, teeth cleaning and other personal care, but also cooking, making a hot drink, shopping and managing finances – even driving and gardening.

Interestingly, one of the criteria that divides mild cognitive impairment (MCI) from dementia is considered to be the ability to carry out ADLs. Of course, someone who has a disability may be unable to do some of these ADLs, and if you are an older person, it may take you longer to carry out some ADLs than it did in the past. If, however, you have no physical disability or temporary injury and you have managed to do all your ADLs in the past, then a developing inability to carry out some or all of them is a matter for concern.

The inability to carry out ADLs can develop slowly – so slowly that it is only when you stop and think back to some time in the past that you may become aware that things have changed and you cannot do the things you used to. Perhaps, for example, someone who was previously an enthusiastic cook gets in a muddle one day and cannot follow a recipe or confuses the timing of the cooking of meat and vegetables so is unable to serve all the components of a meal together on time. If it happens once we may put it down to tiredness, stress or a minor infection that affects the ability to cope. If it starts to happen more often, a partner or family member may begin to assist or may even take over the cooking of more complicated dishes. For some time the person concerned can still carry out simple cooking tasks such as putting together breakfast dishes or making a cup of tea or coffee. A couple can jog along like this without consciously realizing that things have changed quite considerably.

Or possibly the housework tasks begin to cause difficulty. If two people live together, certain tasks tend to fall into the remit of one or the other as a general rule. One person always does the vacuuming or changes the bed linen and does the laundry; the other washes up and takes the rubbish out to the dustbin. If one member of a domestic partnership lets their routine tasks lapse, the other may not notice for a while. When they do notice they may offer to help out with the tasks they do not usually do. After a while this 'helping out' becomes routine, and perhaps after a few months it is realized that only one person is now undertaking all of the domestic tasks.

In this context we are not discussing any rearrangement that may have to be made if one member of the household has an accident or illness and becomes unable to carry out their usual routine because of injury or fatigue due solely to this. If you break your leg no one would expect you to climb a ladder to decorate the ceiling until your leg is fully healed. If you are (for example) undergoing chemotherapy, which causes bouts of exhaustion, your family would naturally rally round and help you with mundane tasks until you are fit again. An inability to manage ADLs that is permanent and not caused by any illness or incident is a cause for concern.

As we get older many of us consider using a helping hand for tasks that are becoming more onerous. This is only natural and not to be confused with an inability to manage ADLs on a daily basis. So if, for example, a keen gardener finds that the hedge cutting is becoming too difficult and time consuming and employs a gardener to do this whilst still enjoying carrying out routine tasks in the garden, this would not be considered a cause for concern. Rather, it would be considered a prudent and wise step. If the same formerly keen gardener ceases to potter around the garden and makes excuses about this, begins sowing a row of plants and wanders off in the middle of the task, becomes unable to name the plants or 'forgets' to do the weeding of a prize flowerbed, we are seeing a different picture.

As stated, one of the criteria that doctors use (and it is not the only one) to distinguish between the early stages of dementia in a patient and a designation of MCI is the continuing ability to carry out ADLs. So if you have MCI, you are still able to carry out your ADLs even if it takes you longer than previously or you have had to modify how you do them. The question is, then, can we use the action of carrying out ADLs to help our MCI?

I think you can.

'Use it or lose it'

What exactly does this overused phrase mean? Many people take it to mean that we should keep 'exercising' the brain by doing crosswords, suduko or other paper puzzles. A recent piece of research reported in the *British Medical Journal*[1] appeared to debunk this idea, but then most experts have known all along that doing puzzles and brain games only succeeds in making you better at doing puzzles and brain games – and then only better at doing the ones you have been used to doing.

It is true, however, that if you cease to practise any activity you will become less able to do it – your ability will become 'rusty', to use a common phrase. Most people know the adage that if you learn to swim or ride a bicycle you do not lose that ability, and this is true. Your brain has learned the pattern of activity required to carry out the action. Even if you do not then ride a bicycle for several decades, you are still able to pick it up again very quickly. This is because your brain learned the motor sequence and response originally, and that information is still encoded in its synapses and circuits – it just needs a bit of refinement. If you have not ridden a bicycle for a long time, you will find that, although you can still do all the right actions and maintain your balance, your skills are slower, your confidence may be affected and your energy (meaning the length of time you can cycle) is less.

Test the truth of this by considering any of your friends (or perhaps yourself) who regularly use a sat nav in the car. People who are overly reliant on the sat nav become unable to drive to a destination without it. Indeed, I have a colleague who regularly drives to my house (maybe five or six times a year). On every occasion she calls to ask me beforehand for the postcode to put into her sat nav. When I once pointed out that having driven from her house to mine several times she must now be familiar with the route, she explained that she was quite unable to recall the route because she 'let the sat nav direct her' and made no effort to notice any road features or routes.

It is important that we reconsider what is meant by the phrase 'use it or lose it' and expand it to include all our daily life – all our 'activities of daily living', in fact – that is, all the things we do on a daily or weekly basis to continue living our everyday lives.

As we slow down with age it is natural to decrease certain activities. Things that attracted us when we were young may no longer seem so interesting now (climbing mountains or running marathons). Physical abilities decrease, and we naturally reduce the more energetic activities in favour of things that take less energy and effort (watching cricket instead of playing it, perhaps). Our social circle might grow smaller, and without even realizing that we are doing so, we make less effort to meet new people or to expand our circle of acquaintances and friends. We may make time-saving changes to our routines. We might give up certain hobbies and pastimes as they seem less attractive or involve compromises in our relationships with others (for example, we might consider that attending football practice every week is not worth the complaints we receive from our left-at-home partner). All these changes are natural and common in older people, and I make no suggestion that there is anything intrinsically wrong in falling into a slower pace of life.

Everyday matters

I am going to suggest that you can take action to help your MCI through the activities you do every day. You do not need to join a club, go to the gym, take up classes or begin to do puzzles and games unless these are things that you already enjoy. Let us review again the suggestion I made in Chapter 1 to picture how the brain copes with neural loss.

When explaining dementia in my training sessions I often liken what happens to the experience of driving around a town. If a road is closed (perhaps due to road works), traffic will be diverted down a different route. Should you be taking this alternative route and find it congested due to, say, a traffic accident, you might turn off down a side road if you know the area and find your way to your destination by taking a series of diversions that do not constitute a direct route, but nevertheless get you where you plan to go. When areas of the brain are damaged, the thinking, planning and actioning process might need to take a longer route than the direct way, and the brain is very good at using such diversions to get where it needs to go. Mostly we are unaware of this 'diversion' process.

Now, suppose we get used to the diversion we have taken – maybe it seems to be an easier, less congested route. We may decide to always take this route in future. After a whilst we may forget the old route altogether because we no longer travel that way. If we are forced to take the old route we may feel a bit apprehensive about doing so because we are no longer used to it. We might perhaps put off using the old route because of this nervousness or ask someone else to drive us on that occasion. Such apprehension can build up in our mind to the extent that we refuse ever to take the old route again. It becomes a big 'no-no' and we have been forced to restrict our lives due to this fear of changing route.

Of course, I am not literally talking about driving here, although we will discuss the action of driving a car later in this chapter. I am just using this idea of roadworks and diversions to show how we can imagine the brain working and in turn to picture how failing to exercise the brain can gradually narrow our choices of action and restrict our viewpoint to the extent that the brain is unable to conceive of an alternative 'route' and is unable to use that route even if it is available.

No, what I am suggesting is that you continue to do the everyday things you do every day. Resist the temptation to avoid doing something because it seems 'such an effort'. Effort is good for you and for your brain. When you think about some everyday task, do not think that it is going to be hard or boring or tiresome. Believe that every time you do this task it is keeping your brain fit and lively. Doing the things you are used to doing is important. If you let someone else or something else (such as a machine) take over the task, you are allowing your brain to lose a little of its ability to function.

Remember the story about my friend who is 'hooked' on using her sat nav? If you always let the sat nav tell you where to go, your brain will stop trying to work out the route. If the brain stops doing something for long enough it loses the ability to do that thing. The neural pathways atrophy.

Of course, this does not mean that you should never use something that helps you to complete a task faster or more easily. Why wash dishes when the dishwasher will do the task easily and well? But do not forget how to wash dishes by hand, or you may find yourself in trouble when the dishwasher needs repairing.

Let us look at some everyday actions – 'activities of daily living', if you like the term – and see how we can use these actions and tasks to help our brain keep active and lively.

Household tasks

Everyone who lives independently (that is, not in residential care) has to carry out household tasks on a daily basis – things like vacuuming the carpets, washing up, doing the laundry, cooking meals and taking out the rubbish. These tasks are part of independent living. They show to others that we can function without help. If you are hospitalized and are elderly and live alone, before you are discharged from hospital the social care team will make sure that you can get around your own home, dress, undress and make a simple hot drink and snack. If you are unable to do these things they may consider that you are unable to function independently.

Many of these household tasks are mundane and even boring to carry out, but consider how each task uses our brain.

Washing up

Washing up involves the brain in *sorting* the various items to be washed, *calculating* the heat of the water and the amount of detergent used, *analysing* the order in which items should be washed (cleaner items before heavily used, greasy items, for example), using *hand–eye coordination* in order to move dishes from the sink to the drainer without breaking them, and *ordering* the entire process – washing, drying, putting away. Even if you use a dishwashing machine for the actual washing up, you will have to arrange items, charge the dishwasher with powder or rinse aid, and select the correct programme, and you will have to unload and put items away later.

Vacuuming or cleaning floors

For this task we need to assess the area to be cleaned (a quick whip round with the vacuum cleaner or a major moving-the-furniture effort), *understand* how to use the machine, *work out* the procedure to ensure the whole room is cleaned, *remember* what parts have been cleaned and what parts still need to be done, assess the state of the finished job and redo any bits left out.

Taking out the rubbish

Our brain needs to *acknowledge* that the rubbish needs clearing, *assess* what is rubbish and what is clutter that simply needs putting away, *sort* the rubbish into what can be recycled and into what container (this can be challenging in some areas) and use *hand–eye coordination and balance* to carry the rubbish outside to its receptacles. We would also need to be aware of the rubbish collection date and coordinate our efforts with this date.

Laundry

Managing the household laundry uses again the ability to *assess* the amount of dirty laundry stacking up, the need to *sort* the items to be washed into suitable wash loads, *understand* how the washing machine works, *use* the correct amount and type of washing powder, *manage* the task in the correct order (collect, sort, wash, dry, iron) and *sort the finished articles into categories* and put them away in the right places at the end of the process.

When you assess simple household tasks in this way you become aware of how many abilities you are using just to carry out these ADLs. It seems amazing that your brain is not exhausted just by everyday living!

Now consider that by asking someone else to do one of these tasks you are depriving your brain of exercise. Better still, be aware that every time you actually carry out one of these mundane activities you are strengthening your brain's neural pathways. This is not an exaggeration. People who have dementia gradually lose the ability to do all these things: to assess, calculate, manage, understand, order and remember.

So, one of the first and easiest things you can do if you have MCI and want to help yourself – that is, to try to arrest any progress to dementia – is to carry on with your daily routine tasks. It doesn't matter if it takes you a little longer to do what you have always done, or if you have to concentrate more to achieve the result you want. Remember that each task exercises the brain.

Shopping

We all know that the internet has revolutionized our lives – and perhaps this is most noticeable when it comes to shopping. Many of us find ourselves saying, if we cannot find an item when in the shops, 'I'll buy it online'. Even if you are one of the very few who never shops online, the internet will be affecting how you shop. Major stores now do all their stock-taking via the web and will be able to tell you that 'Our store in such and such a town has that item if you wish to go there'. Or they will offer to order an item for you to collect at a later date. They are able to do this because they can order online and take your details on their computer to make sure of notifying you when the item comes in.

Some older people get their weekly or monthly bulk shop delivered, having ordered what they want online. In some ways this harks back to how our parents and grandparents lived. My mother used to drop her 'order book' into the local grocer's shop each week and the items she ordered were delivered neatly packed in a cardboard box later in the week. Sometimes, these days, it is a helpful son or daughter who 'goes online' and puts in the order, and a friendly delivery driver will come up with the goods on the specified date.

Shopping online may be detrimental to the high street, as the media often tells us, but it is convenient and useful, and arguably uses the brain just as much as walking around numerous shops and comparing actual goods as opposed to pictures of goods. Indeed, it may be very good 'brain exercise' to try to establish whether a particular garment or item of food is exactly what is required. To find out more than the basic picture shows, you usually have to 'drill down' through a description, various sub-headings such as 'ingredients' or 'fabric content', and sometimes even click through to find out via the 'reviews' what experience other customers have had of the product.

Whether you choose to shop online or by actually walking around the shops is not the point here. What is important is that you continue to do your own shopping. If you have a physical problem that prevents you getting to the shops, then at least make the effort to choose your own purchases. Grocery shopping online is, in fact, very simple

– the supermarkets make sure that this is so. Even if you feel that you are not computer-'savvy', perhaps you could learn to manage this. If you must allow a relative or friend to manage your online shopping for you, be sure not to delegate the all-important selection and decision-making. Write your own lists and discuss them with your handy 'computer expert'; don't just accept the same grocery order every week or – worse still – allow someone else to decide what you will eat in the coming days.

If you are able to go out shopping, this is a very useful thing to do, even if only for certain purchases. The travel to the shops, choosing what shops to visit, examining and comparing goods and interacting with shop workers and other customers is stimulating for your brain – and walking around is good for your physical health too.

Whichever way you choose (or perhaps are forced) to shop, at least remember to do as much as you can yourself.

Driving

Driving deserves a separate heading because it can sometimes be a real cause for concern – not only for the driver, but also for younger relatives or friends who may feel that you should no longer be driving. In my work I frequently have conversations with people who have a huge reluctance to consult their doctor even if they are worried about their memory because they are convinced that 'the doctor will stop me driving'. This book is concerned with MCI and not specifically with dementia, but it might reassure those people I have mentioned above to know that as the law stands at present, a diagnosis of dementia does not automatically bar someone from driving.

There is an interesting two-sided view here. Many people, as they grow older, dislike driving more than they used to. Partly this is due to an increase in traffic on the roads, partly to the knowledge of slower reactions or problems with vision or flexibility (driving a car involves quite a bit of body movement, particularly if manoeuvring the car when parking, etc.), and partly this is due to the sheer awareness of potential danger. Very few people like to admit this growing dislike, but you may find that you are avoiding driving for long distances or in areas that you do not know well. If someone offers to drive you, it may be that you are more likely to accept the offer than in the past. Perhaps you do not avoid driving but you just find yourself more apprehensive when contemplating a long or complicated journey.

On the other hand, nobody wants to be stopped from driving. Many people resist vigorously when younger family members suggest, for example, that perhaps they should give up their driving licence. If asked, most people would say that the reason they resist giving up their licence is because they want 'to keep their independence'. Indeed, the problem of poor public transport, closure of local shops and amenities, coupled with a reduced vigour and the physical trials of age all mean that living without a car can be very restricting.

So how do you deal with these two contrasting aspects of the problem?

First, try to remove your feelings from the equation. The suggestion that you may find driving more difficult or that you may no longer be safe to drive is not a reflection on your worth as a person. Nor does it necessarily imply that you are becoming infirm. It is simply someone else's opinion. If you can review the matter coolly and without emotion, you will be able to make the right decisions about driving.

Second, whether you feel more nervous yourself or whether someone close to you is suggesting that you are unfit to drive, get an unbiased opinion. There are a number of options to do this. The Royal Society for the Prevention of Accidents (RoSPA) offers a driving assessment for people who want an honest opinion. It is not a 'test' and they do not report the result of your assessment to anyone else. They do, however, offer an unbiased opinion of your driving skills and give you a one-to-one report after the assessment, together with suggestions to help you drive more safely in future.[2] In some counties in the UK, Advanced Driving Schools offer a similar service.

Third, take sensible precautions. The RoSPA website offers a number of safety tips for older drivers that are summed up here as follows:

- Make sure that your general health does not disqualify you from driving.
- Have regular vision checks to make sure you are safe to drive.
- Keep your car roadworthy and consider changing your car for a simpler or more comfortable model, if necessary.

- Avoid driving in bad weather conditions.
- Plan your route to avoid driving on roads you find problematic.
- Make other transport arrangements for long or difficult journeys.

These suggestions are wise options for any older person who wishes to continue to drive. Driving is a mechanical skill that is 'hard-wired' into the brain, and many older people are actually safer and more competent drivers than younger people, so if you are happy to drive and still feel confident, then by all means continue to do so. If, on the other hand, you are less confident and would prefer to avoid driving, then look at all the other options available to you. We consider some of these in Chapter 7.

Socializing

Studies have found that a varied social life, plenty of different interests and mixing with a wide variety of people are considered, along with a broad educational experience, to be protective factors against dementia, but it is sometimes hard to distinguish cause and effect. Does an outgoing and sociable person avoid dementia because of their varied social life, or is it that someone who is outgoing and sociable is less likely to become demented because of their personality? We know that people with dementia tend to become less sociable and to avoid going out and about and mixing with those they do not know well. But we also know that dementia takes many years to develop to the extent that symptoms become obvious. The question has to be, is the reluctance to socialize a very early sign of dementia?

If family are asked about social habits, they may say that their relative has 'always been a bit of a loner' or 'has never enjoyed parties' or 'is not the type to join clubs', but it can be hard for family to think back far enough to establish whether being unsociable is an actual character trait or a tendency that has developed recently. Children talking about their elderly parents may give a very inaccurate account because in their early years they will not have been mature enough to analyse their parents' characters.

Whether you are 'sociable' or not it is likely that you do mix with others, speak to people such as neighbours, go out shopping or attend to tradespeople, as all these things are necessary simply to exist in society. So, rather than talking about 'being sociable' we ought, perhaps, to consider whether there have been changes in your normal social intercourse. For example, have you started avoiding answering the front door or the telephone when previously you would have done this as a matter of course? Do you ask others to attend to chores that require you to approach and speak to strangers – for example, if you need to make enquiries at a bank or post office? Do you always frequent familiar shops where they know what your requirements are likely to be?

There may be good reasons why you have changed your social habits if you have done so. Perhaps your hearing has deteriorated and you find it hard to understand what others are saying. Or you may find it hard to get around due to a physical problem so you are not able to go out and about as much as you previously did. But problems like this can be overcome for those who still want to enjoy their usual occupations. If, on the other hand, you are actually choosing not to pursue your usual occupations or to carry out common everyday actions that you formerly did, this is a matter of concern.

If you have MCI, you may be aware of the reasons that you are beginning to change your social habits. You may find it more difficult to follow the rules of a game you play regularly (like bridge or golf), and so you don't play so often. Or perhaps you find yourself forgetting the names of people you meet on a daily basis so you go out of your way to avoid meeting them to avoid embarrassment. You may find it more difficult to find your way to new places when driving and so you try not to go anywhere new. Possibly you get confused when shopping and forget some items you were supposed to buy, so in future you refuse to shop alone. All these are common examples of everyday occasions when MCI may affect your social behaviour.

You may be asking what you should do if some or all of these examples of avoiding everyday social interactions apply to you. Perhaps you are asking yourself whether it matters if you make changes to your social routine to avoid situations you may find difficult.

I suggest that you remember that *if you don't use it, you lose it*. Every time you make an excuse to avoid a situation that seems difficult to you, you are giving your brain a 'get-out', a way to forget how to act in this situation. Each time you avoid a situation it becomes harder to negotiate it the next time it occurs, until eventually you will become unable to cope with this social occasion at all.

What can you do if you are aware that you are beginning to avoid social occasions because of potential confusion? Enlist the help of someone you trust to ease your way. If you have a calm, steady person with you who can help you negotiate your fears and give you confidence in a social situation, this can make a difference, although you don't want to become reliant on this person – rather, you want them to help you to ease your way back to your former confident self.

Another way to tackle this problem is to take smaller steps. If, for example, you have found yourself panicking because you get confused during a trip to the shops, find a quiet time to go shopping. Write yourself a short list of items to buy and think about the route to the shops and what you need to take with you – money and a shopping bag, perhaps.

If you get confused doing a regular hobby like playing bridge or golf, confide in a friend or game partner and ask them to help you. Or you could elect to play only with people you know well and in venues you know well. (But remember, do not stop playing.) You could play shorter matches or withdraw from competitions but still play in 'friendlies' where your competence is less critical to a team.

If you find yourself reluctant to go to social events because you dislike driving after dark or parking in an awkward venue, try to find out if anyone can offer you a lift. People are often pleased to do this as it is common to dislike 'arriving alone', so you may actually be doing someone a favour by asking. You can always offer to help with fuel costs.

If you have MCI, you may find that some ADLs become harder for you, but the important thing – the difference between MCI and dementia – is that you can still do them. Remember that it is important that you do still do them. Take them more slowly, put systems in place to make them easier for you, but continue to do them. The more you carry out activities, the more your brain continues to lay down the pathways that allow you to continue to do them.

Key points

- Activities of daily living are the things you do every day.
- It is easy to stop doing things when they become more difficult to carry out.
- Doing any action less makes it harder to do.
- By all means find easier ways to do everyday things, but do not give up doing them.
- Even doing simple things like household tasks and shopping keeps the brain active.
- Practise safer driving techniques.
- Keep up your social contacts and your leisure interests.

Endnotes

1   Staff, R.J., Hogan, M.J., Williams, D.S. and Whalley, L.J. (2018) 'Intellectual engagement and cognitive ability in later life (the "use it or lose it" conjecture): Longitudinal, prospective study.' *BMJ 363*, k4925, doi:10.1136/bmj.k4925.
2   See www.rospa.com/road-safety/advice/drivers/older

Chapter 5

Factors that May Benefit Cognition

Although we are still not certain of the cause or causes of dementia, much more is now known about the individual risk factors – the factors that may make you more likely to develop cognitive problems. It follows that those things that raise the risk of developing dementia are also likely to raise the risk of mild cognitive impairment (MCI). It is thought that this higher risk is due to a combination of genetic and environmental factors. Research has shown that we can affect environmental factors by making changes to our lifestyle and making the right choices in life. We touched on some of these in Chapter 3, and in this chapter we will examine the various risk factors for dementia and look at how we can affect these with particular regard to MCI.

Factors (with our present state of knowledge) that can make a difference are:

- diet and nutrition
- exercise

- social life and networks
- increasing brain plasticity
- reducing stress
- addressing certain health problems
- getting enough sleep.

Diet and nutrition

Chapter 3 included a discussion on just what is and what is not a 'good healthy diet', and it was emphasized that opinions are constantly changing in this regard. For example, since the 1990s it has been taken as a 'truth' that we should all be eating a low-fat diet for the health of our hearts. But recently this supposed 'truth' has been called into question and the suggestion now is that fat – the 'right kind of fat' – is actually vital for good health. Many books have been written about diet and a great deal of research has been done to investigate whether a certain food or foods will make a difference in various disease states. Unfortunately, we still do not have any definitive answers about whether certain foods are of benefit for cognition. The general advice is that a heart-healthy diet is also a brain-healthy diet, but as noted above, even what constitutes a 'heart-healthy diet' is being called into question.

The media often talk about so-called 'superfoods', which, if consumed, will have a dramatic affect on our health. Alas, it usually transpires that the benefit can only be recognized if we eat huge amounts of these individual foods and avoid many others.

The one thing most experts are agreed on is that it is generally unhealthy to exclude any one food element from our diet unless we have a proven ailment caused by that food (for example, people who suffer from coeliac disease have to avoid eating gluten; others should not exclude this food group). The one exception to this rule is sugar – most experts agree that sugar is of no benefit nutritionally and may be both harmful and addictive. Interestingly, many people with a diagnosis of dementia have an increased appetite for sweet things and, unless prevented, may eat sweet things to the exclusion of other food items.

The best advice to follow is to consume a good varied diet including all the food groups – that is, protein, carbohydrates and fat – and to ensure an adequate intake of vitamins found in fruit and vegetables. There is no evidence to show that food supplements are harmful if taken in the recommended amounts and so, if you feel better when you consume a food supplement, then by all means continue to take it. Be sure, of course, that it does not interfere with any prescribed medication you may be taking.

Exercise

Studies have shown that aerobic exercise, undertaken regularly, actually increases brain volume,[1] and it is now believed that the beneficial effects of aerobic exercise have a direct effect on brain health. Your doctor is therefore likely to advise you that exercise benefits not only your heart and cardiovascular system, but also your brain.

Many people are put off by the suggestion to exercise more because they have visions of Lycra-clad enthusiasts sweating it out in the local gym or pounding the pavements on their 'daily run'. However, exercise can take many forms, and the best exercise for you is certainly doing something you enjoy. Although there is no direct evidence to show that exercise undertaken reluctantly is of less benefit than exercise that is enjoyed, it is more likely that you will be motivated to continue to do something you enjoy.

Exercise does not only mean running or doing 'physical jerks' but any activity that involves moving and twisting the body and raising the breathing rate. Therefore, simple activities such as gardening or games such as golf, tennis and bowls count. Even shopping can be seen as exercise if we take the trouble to park the car at a distance from the shops, to lift shopping into the shopping trolley or car boot, and to unload our purchases and pack them away. I am not suggesting, however, that a weekly shopping trip is sufficient exercise for a healthy body and brain!

If you enjoy a regular exercise activity like golf, swimming or walking, then continue doing it. In Chapter 4 I gave some ideas to use if you are finding it difficult to follow the rules of your game or activity, or if lack of confidence is preventing you from doing it as much as you would like. If, however, you do not do any regular physical exercise, think seriously about beginning to do so.

I have pointed out that you do not have to join a gym or buy special clothing or even spend money in order to exercise. If the idea of taking up something such as golf, tennis or bowls attracts you, by all means look into it. Many clubs offer special 'taster sessions' or are open to the general public on certain days, hoping to attract new members, and this is a good way to find out if you would enjoy an activity and – equally important – enjoy mixing with the people taking part.

If you used to have an active hobby in the past such as running or keep fit, judo or badminton, or yoga, consider resuming this because it is likely to have been something you really enjoyed. You may be a bit 'rusty' if you have been out of action for several years, but there are likely to be others in the same situation, and these days there are often local classes at leisure centres or other nearby places that welcome 'returners'.

Consider also activities you may not think of as 'exercise' such as dancing or swimming. There are many forms of dancing, from ballroom dancing to Zumba, and all of them are good for your physical fitness; some research points to them being good for the brain too! Dancing is also a very good social activity and allows you to meet others who have similar tastes. Swimming is an activity many people forget when they talk about exercise, and although it is a 'non-weight bearing' exercise, and so may not be as good for your bone health as some other forms of exercise, it does keep you active and helps with your breathing and general fitness.

If none of these suggestions attract you, at least get out and increase the amount of walking you do. Walking is a very good exercise and can be made even better by increasing your pace and choosing routes that include hills or rough ground. If you generally only walk to the local shops or round the block with the dog, there is scope for you to extend this activity by choosing to walk a little further each day; varying your route can help your brain too, as you can read in Chapter 3.

Social life and networks

Having a varied social life, mixing with a variety of people and a broad education and experience are considered to be protective against developing dementia, but some researchers consider instead that sociable and interactive people are less likely to develop dementia because of the kind of person they are. In other words, they think that someone who is sociable and lively has a brain less likely to slide into dementia, rather than suggesting that increasing social activity and meeting new people will prevent dementia irrespective of the kind of person you are.

This is a complicated area and research has not clarified things much. On the one hand, some research such as the Nun Study[2] suggests that personality traits in early and mid-life have strong relationships with the risk of Alzheimer's disease. In this interesting long-term study, David Snowdon studied the lifestyle, diet and exercise habits of 678 nuns over a period of many years, and the study included the nuns' donation of their brains after death for research. Snowdon's examination of autobiographical essays written by the nuns on joining the sisterhood seemed to indicate that a lack of complexity and fluency in written ability in early life predicted the risk of developing dementia in old age. But other research seems to indicate that we can decrease the risk of developing dementia by increasing our social interaction.[3]

Whichever of these points of view you believe, it is known that people who are 'loners', who live a solitary and introverted lifestyle, are more likely to be depressed and to avoid social contact. Studies of Cognitive Stimulation

Therapy (CST) – a group social therapy recommended by NICE (National Institute Health and Care Excellence) for people with early stage dementia – indicate that an increase in social interaction in a calm and non-threatening environment increases a feeling of well-being and makes a difference to mood and functioning.[4]

People who have MCI often begin to avoid social occasions and to reject contact with those who are not well known to them because they may feel less confident in social situations. They may also be afraid that they will no longer be able to participate fully in group discussions and activities due to reduced abilities and slower reactions. This can cause embarrassment because if you cannot follow a conversation well, you may think that everyone is noticing your hesitation and difficulty. It is likely, however, that no one is noticing your perceived problem. Generally, when in a group conversation people are more aware of their own contribution and may be thinking about what they will say next rather than noticing if someone else is not joining in as much as usual.

Whether you lean towards the suggestion that a sociable person is less likely to develop dementia or the belief that an active social life protects you from the risk of dementia, it is worth making the effort to continue your social activities and to mix with others as much as possible, even if you have MCI and need some help to do this.

It is probably a good idea not to embark on a new form of activity if you are not feeling very confident, but you can at least continue to engage with others as you have been used to doing: attend clubs, sports or activities you have been attending in the past and try not to avoid social situations purely on the grounds that you may feel less comfortable than before. So, if you are a member of a group or club, continue to attend meetings. If you are feeling less confident than previously, you may like to give up extra responsibilities such as sitting on a committee or holding a particular voluntary post in the club organization, but you can still attend meetings and join in events. If you need a little help in some areas, you may be surprised to find that many others do as well, and that there are plenty of people who will happily provide that help. Here are some examples given to me by clients (of course, names and identities have been changed or masked in these examples):

Beth was a keen member of a local church choir and attended weekly meetings without fail. When she started claiming to 'feel sick' before meetings, her husband wondered what was wrong. It turned out that she was worrying about parking her car in the cramped church car park. Beth's husband asked around and another choir member offered to give Beth a lift each week. This meant that she could attend without worrying about the car parking.

Michael was a member of a social/charitable club where each member took turns to be president of the club for a year. As his year of presidency approached, Michael became very worried that he would not be able to cope with the pressures of being president, and he told his family that he planned to resign from the club because he had lost interest in its aims. Fortunately, one of Michael's sons suspected that there was more involved than a simple loss of interest, and he managed to have a heart-to-heart with his dad and discover his fears. The present president of the club was approached and with the agreement of him and his committee, Michael was able to side-step the presidency and continue to attend as an ordinary member.

Doreen enjoyed the 'knit and natter' group to which she belonged and indeed, it was the centre of her life. Her daughter became worried when Doreen started avoiding going to the weekly meetings. Eventually she found out that Doreen was finding the more complicated knitting patterns hard to do, and one or two club members had made some unfortunate remarks about her muddled knitting. Doreen's daughter also enjoyed knitting and so she began attending the group with her mother, sitting with her and shielding her from the more unpleasant members. She also had a word with the club organizer, and these two measures meant that Doreen continued enjoying the company and the club.

Dave enjoyed playing golf and much of his social life centred round the golf club. However, he began finding that he was getting rather slow at calculating the score and also had difficulty orientating himself on the course. Other club members complained about his slowness and this made him decide to resign from the club. However, a close friend who was also a club member intervened.

He agreed to keep score when he played with Dave. He also suggested that if Dave still had difficulties as time went on, he could remain as a 'social' member only so that he could still enjoy the company of other club members and could continue to use the driving range even if he did not play matches.

What does this mean in terms of everyday life?

- Keep attending any clubs or activities you have always enjoyed. See the examples above for ideas about how to adapt if you feel less confident.
- Engage with friends and family as much as you can. These are the people who know you best. Tell them if you feel you have difficulties so that they can help and support you. Usually we find that we can be more relaxed amongst our close friends and family, and our difficulties are consequently less obvious.
- Don't be afraid to ask for help or support if you need it. Don't feel embarrassed. It may surprise you to find that others have had the same difficulties – you are probably not the first. It is also true that many people are keen to help others and there may be areas where you can offer help in return.

Reducing stress

Some stress is good for the brain and the body. A certain amount of the 'right' stress keeps us lively and alert. But chronic stress – being in a situation where you feel you have no control over what happens why or when – exerts a great strain on both the body and brain. We all know the situation where someone asks us a routine question ('What is your phone number?') and our mind goes blank. Or perhaps you have had to contact someone urgently and their contact details go straight out of your head. This situation is caused by momentary stress. Indeed, we know that if we can take a few minutes to calm down and remove ourselves from the stress of the moment, the information is again at our fingertips.

If stress can cause this to happen to someone with no obvious cognitive problems, think about how much worse the stressful experience may be for someone who is already cognitively challenged.

Any kind of stressful situation is likely to make cognition worse and chronic stress may lead to chronic cognitive problems. Try to avoid becoming over-stressed. Plan ahead if you are going to have a busy day or if you are going into a situation that is new to you. Check out your route, decide what clothes you will wear ahead of time, buy anything you need (such as gifts) in good time, get up early so that you do not have to rush, and leave in plenty of time if you have a journey. These are all good and sensible precautions that will prevent you becoming over-stressed.

Many people benefit from calming techniques, and even if you haven't thought about it before, consider incorporating some of these into your life. There are many different forms of calming techniques and you will be sure to find something that suits you if you investigate. For example, there is simple meditation, and many people find this works for them. There are forms of exercise that incorporate mind-calming moves such as yoga and tai chi. These exercise and mind-calming methods are both easily adapted to be used by older people. A well-publicized calming technique currently in vogue is mindfulness – the action of simply being in the here and now without allowing yourself to worry about the past or the future.

There are classes in all these calming techniques and many are available at very small cost in your local area. If you do not wish to join a 'class' you can buy books that will guide you or you can find YouTube videos free on the internet.

You may think that this kind of calming behaviour is not for you, especially if in the past you have associated it with 'alternative' thinking. It is important here to be open-minded and prepared to try things out. If you do not like a particular method of stress release, you can stop using it. Nothing is written in stone and no method works for everyone. It is likely that you will find some method of calming technique that will work for you.

General health – physical and mental

It is easy to consider that our mind and our body are two separate things and that nothing we do physically will affect our mental capacity, but current medical thinking believes otherwise. Our general physical health can also impact our mental health. Chronic physical problems can result in clinical depression.

Some physical illnesses have a known association with dementia and cognitive problems. For example, having type 2 diabetes (maturity onset) is known to raise the risk of developing dementia. A raised risk does not mean that you will definitely develop dementia, but it makes sense to make every effort to reduce risk factors if you already have MCI.

If you have diabetes follow your doctor's advice and keep control of your blood sugar levels. New research seems to indicate that in some cases diabetes can be reversed by making changes to lifestyle and diet.[5] Since diabetes carries many risks in addition to the raised risk of developing dementia – it can affect eyesight, circulation and other health issues – any offer of remission is worth considering (although doctors insist that a reversal is a remission and not a cure). The main factor seems to be weight loss. You can ask at your doctor's surgery or ask your diabetic nurse for information about reversing diabetes, but you should not stop taking any prescription medication without agreement from your doctor.

Hearing loss

Hearing loss is another risk factor for dementia. It is known that someone with reduced hearing has a raised risk of developing dementia. It is not known whether attending to the loss of hearing by using hearing aids reduces the risk. However, social isolation is also a risk factor for developing dementia, and reduced hearing means increased social isolation. Someone who has difficulty in hearing and joining in with conversations or in making sense of what is going on around them becomes less inclined to take part in social groups. It is sensible to have your hearing checked regularly and to use hearing aids if these are prescribed. It can be difficult to get used to hearing aids, but most people who persist say that the benefits are worth the effort.

Depression

Depression is common in older people and is often ignored or dismissed as being one of the problems of 'getting old', but depression can lead to social isolation. Depression is treatable and you should consult your doctor and not dismiss any symptoms as being due to increasing age. Depression can also lead to sleep problems.

Sleep problems

Recent research indicates that getting enough sleep is an important factor in maintaining cognition at optimal levels.[6] There is an increased awareness that we all need to sleep properly for around eight hours a night in order to function well. Older people need slightly less sleep than younger people, but a good night's sleep is still essential.

There are many things you can do to improve your sleep pattern without resorting to medication:

- Avoid electronic devices for at least an hour before retiring; this includes eReaders, phones and tablets as well as laptops.

- Do not keep electronic devices in your bedroom.
- Lower the lighting in the bedroom immediately before you sleep.
- Ensure the bedroom is dark and quiet: some people find ear plugs and sleep masks useful.
- Bedroom temperature should be cool (not cold) and bed coverings should be lightweight but adequate.
- Some people find that keeping the bedroom uncluttered helps to calm them at bedtime.
- Do not watch TV in bed before sleeping.
- Do not read exciting books before sleeping.
- Do not eat too soon before bedtime, but avoid going to bed feeling hungry.
- Some people find that sleeping in a separate bed (or a separate room) from a partner helps them to sleep better.
- Go to bed at a regular time and if you wake in the night try not to get up – do not switch on lights unless strictly necessary.
- If you need to use the toilet during the night, try to ensure that you are disturbed as little as possible.
- Work out a soothing 'back to sleep' ritual you can use if you do wake up. Some people count sheep or recite a boring exercise such as the times tables; some people have a mental 'picture' they can call on that is soothing; some people play music in their heads.
- Lavender oil and other scents can work for some people when sprayed on pillows or rubbed onto the skin.

Education and learning (brain plasticity)

Those who have had a good education (at least 12 years' schooling) are less likely to develop dementia.[7] It is not known exactly why a poor or limited education raises the risk, but the most likely reason is thought to be that early education increases brain plasticity – that is, the ability of the brain to find new ways to manipulate data and solve problems. It used to be thought that once you reached adulthood the brain could not form new neurons and the limit of plasticity had been reached. However, it is now known that new neurons continue to form, even into old age. If we have not had the benefit of a thorough early education, it is not too late at any time of life to improve on our early experience. There are many daytime and evening classes available at small cost or even free. If this kind of 'formal' education does not appeal, we can – any of us – learn through using libraries, internet facilities (there are many free learning resources online) and informal groups such as the University of the Third Age (U3A).

Extending the brain does not have to mean 'schoolwork'. Taking up a new sport or hobby, learning another language through conversation with a foreign national, planning new routes for walks using maps and GPS systems, exploring new areas of the countryside or learning a skill like typing or driving are all ways we can encourage the brain to develop, whatever our age.

Lifestyle - smoking, alcohol, drugs

Some suggestions for better health are self-evident. All the evidence now clearly suggests that cigarette smoking is bad for your health, and mental health is no exception to this. If you are a smoker, try to quit. There is currently plenty of help available to support you in this.

The evidence for drinking alcohol is more equivocal. At present most advice seems to suggest that moderate alcohol intake does no harm, and may even be beneficial. The term 'moderate' is difficult to define because the advised limits on units of alcohol are rather arbitrary. However, if you find that your drinking habits make you feel ill either at the time or the 'morning after', this suggests that you are overdoing it. It should go without saying that drinking and driving is potentially bad for your health (considering the potential for accidents) as well as against the law.

Illegal drugs are illegal because they are considered to be harmful. There is some suggestion that drug taking in the past can affect your health as you age,[8] but we cannot go back and re-live our lives to eliminate any harm done in the past, so it is pointless worrying about this now.

Medication

Older people are likely to be taking more than one prescription drug, and most people assume that the doctor has ensured that none of the drugs they take interact with each other. I am constantly amazed when speaking to my clients that large numbers of people seem to take medication when prescribed by the doctor even if they do not know what the benefit is supposed to be. Many people do not even know why they are taking the pills they take each day. Few of them ever check whether the drug will affect their mood or their thinking ability. But a number of drugs given to older people can affect cognition, so if you have MCI, always check with your doctor to see if this may be a side effect of any drugs you have been prescribed.

The doctor should, in theory, check any prescription at the time of prescribing to ensure that it does not 'clash' with any other drugs prescribed. In practice, time constraints may prevent this.

If you are at all worried about interactions between any of the medications you have been prescribed, first check with your doctor. You can also easily check yourself using any of various websites if you are computer-literate. You should not stop taking medication if something you read online suggests an interaction between medications that you have been prescribed, but instead take this information back to your doctor and ask for a clear explanation. It will not alienate your doctor if you explain that you do not understand all the implications and need clear advice.

One sensible practice is to be aware of any new symptoms that arise soon after taking a new prescription medicine. In such a case, if there is no other obvious cause, it is very likely that the new symptoms are a side effect of the medication. Make a note of these symptoms and check with your pharmacist or doctor. Many people do not bother to read the explanatory leaflet that comes with their medication. I have heard people say that they avoid reading the leaflet because they will be worried about side effects.

It is important to take careful note of what the leaflet says. If 10 per cent of people taking a particular drug are likely to experience a side effect, this means that 90 per cent (that is 90 out of every 100 people taking the drug) will *not* experience the side effect. Therefore, the odds are that you will not experience this particular side effect.

Sometimes any side effects are less important than the action of the drug. You need to be sensible and careful with any medication, prescription or otherwise.

A good practice for anyone with MCI is to register with and use only one pharmacist for all prescriptions. Pharmacists are usually meticulous about checking drug interactions. You can also ask the pharmacist if you are worried about interactions or side effects even if you feel unable to question the doctor.

Keep up with new research

You don't have to be a scientist to be aware of new research about cognitive impairment: the media is full of the latest news stories about 'a cure for Alzheimer's' or 'the cause of memory loss'. If you have MCI and are serious about helping yourself and doing all you can to prevent a downward spiral into a dementia diagnosis, keeping abreast of new research is worthwhile. The important thing to do is to read the news stories carefully and wherever possible trace back to the source – usually a newly published research paper. Not all claims of a breakthrough bear investigation. Frequently you will find that the news story is based on a study of mice in the laboratory or is simply a re-hashed version of some previous research. It takes patience and some expertise to read research papers intelligently, but look carefully at any 'abstract' that should give the key points in understandable language. Most often you will find that the conclusion of the research is expressed much more cautiously than the newspaper headlines suggest.

However, if you do find a new research conclusion that looks promising, it is worth finding out all you can. Don't just expect your doctor to be able to give you the answers. Doctors are so busy that new research may have passed them by. You will have to become your own expert. As you get used to following up stories about new 'miracle cures' you will begin to learn the trustworthy names and the journals that publish worthwhile research. Always ask yourself whether the answers and conclusions of the research actually demonstrate new knowledge or facts.

Remember that when you have MCI, the person who is most concerned in improving your chances of not developing dementia is you (and possibly your nearest and dearest). You will soon become an expert in anything that helps your cognition and functioning. If you find that something helps you, then (provided it is legal, of course) use it to improve your life.

Key points

- We still do not know what causes dementia, but we do know some of the 'risk factors'.
- If you have MCI, it is worth addressing any risk factors.

- Aim for optimum health levels, good nutritional status and a varied social life.
- Try to increase your brain plasticity.
- Do not take unnecessary medication and always check with your doctor or pharmacist about side effects that may affect your cognition.
- Take sensible exercise and do not smoke or use recreational drugs.
- Become the expert on what helps you and do not rely on others – doctors or family – to do this for you.

Endnotes

1   Colcombe, S.J., Erickson, K.I., Scalf, P.E., Kim, J.S., *et al.* (2006) 'Aerobic exercise training increases brain volume in aging humans.' *Journals of Gerontology: series A – Biological Sciences and Medical Sciences 61*, 11, 1166–1170.

2   Snowden, D. (2011) Ageing with Grace. *The Nun Study and the science of old age: How we can all live longer, healthier and more vital lives.* London: Fourth Estate.

3   Marioni, R.E., Proust-Lima, C., Amieva, H., Brayne, C., *et al.* (2015) 'Social activity, cognitive decline and dementia risk: A 20-year prospective cohort study.' *BMC Public Health 15*, 1089. Available at https://bmcpublichealthbiomedcentral.com/articles/10.1186/s12889-015-2426-6

4   Livingston, G., Sommerlad, A., Orgeta, V., Costafreda, S.G., *et al.* (2017) 'Dementia prevention, intervention and care.' *The Lancet 390*, 10113.

5   Pierce, M. (2013) 'Type 2 diabetes: Prevention and cure?' *British Journal of General Practice 63*, 607, 60–61. doi:10.3399/bjgp13X661002

6   Yaffe, K., Laffan, A.M., Harrison, S.L., Redline, S., *et al.* (2011) 'Sleep-disordered breathing, hypoxia, and risk of mild cognitive impairment and dementia in older women.' *JAMA 306*, 6, 613–619. doi:10.1001/jama.2011.1115

7   Livingston *et al.* (2017), op cit.

8   Gobbi, G., Atkin, T., Zytynski, T., Wang, S., *et al.* (2019) 'Association of cannabis use in adolescence and risk of depression, anxiety, and suicidality in young adulthood: A systematic review and meta-analysis.' *JAMA Psychiatry 76*, 4, 426–434. doi:10.1001/jamapsychiatry.2018.4500

Chapter 6

Memory Aids

Many people find that their memory needs a little help as they age. It is no disgrace to need memory aids and indeed, if they help you to continue to manage your activities of daily living (ADLs) and to be independent, this can only benefit you. Do not feel that you are 'giving in' or letting yourself down by using a little help. Rather, you are taking sensible and mature action to ensure that you will be less of a burden on others.

Sometimes quite simple options can make a big difference. In this chapter we look at a wide variety of memory aids and other items that can help with spatial problems or general confusion. We also examine what you can do to help yourself if you have a few cognitive problems.

Often the simplest memory aids are the most useful. Just because something is 'the latest thing' does not mean that it is better than what went before. A shopping list written with a pencil and paper is still a shopping list – an aid to the memory. If a younger relative uses his/her smartphone to produce the same shopping list, it doesn't mean it is any more effective. Use the methods that suit you best to help yourself.

As a general rule, do not try to learn something new in order to help your memory. For example, if you have never used computer technology, it is unlikely that trying to learn to use a laptop or tablet (such as an iPad) will be helpful. It is more likely to make you confused and frustrated, so ignore any well-meant attempts on the part of younger relatives to 'bring you up-to-date'. On the other hand, if you are an enthusiastic user of IT and always try to keep up with the latest trend, you may find phone apps and electronic reminders extremely useful.

Diaries and calendars

Diaries and calendars are some of the most basic and also some of the most useful memory aids. Most of us are used to having a calendar to consult or a diary to record appointments. Some people keep a regular 'journal' form of diary in which they write about the day or week just past.

A large-print eye-catching calendar is a most useful thing. Hang it where it will catch your eye and in a place that makes it convenient to use to note appointments or events. To make a calendar useful you will need to develop two habits (if you don't already have them); the first is to note on the calendar everything you want to remember – every appointment, event or regular happening. The second is to look at the calendar regularly. First thing in the morning is a good time for this and at least once later in the day – perhaps late afternoon – to remind yourself of anything happening the next day for which you need to prepare.

In short:

- Buy a calendar and hang it where you will notice it.
- Be sure to write on the calendar all appointments and events on the correct dates.
- Look at the calendar at least twice a day to remind yourself of what you need to recall.

If you prefer and are used to keeping a diary, the same principles apply:

- Buy a diary in the form you have always used. Some people like a large diary they can have open on a hall table; others like something small enough to carry with them. Some people still feel most comfortable with a traditional-style diary that incorporates an address book and other features.
- Be sure to write in your diary all appointments and events on the correct dates.
- Look at diary frequently to remind yourself of upcoming appointments.

If you are used to keeping a 'journal-type' diary, ensure you keep writing it up. It will be immensely useful as a memory aid and will also be a pleasant reminder of the past days and weeks, enabling you to jog your memory about past events. You may be surprised sometimes to read your journal and be reminded of things that have happened and that have slipped your mind. Such a diary will also be a good reminder of the days of the week and seasons, which can blend into one if your life is mundane and you perhaps live alone. So, if you keep a journal-type diary, it is a good thing to read it through at least once every week to remind yourself of what you have been doing.

Alarms

Alarms in whatever form are extremely useful. However good our memory, it is easy to become distracted and to forget timings of different procedures.

There are many kinds of alarm. Everyone is acquainted with the standard alarm clock, although you may be surprised to know that young people hardly ever use such things, preferring to be alerted and reminded via their mobile phone. A standard alarm clock is also fairly limited in that it is generally used for one reminder (such as time to wake up) in every 24 hours, and following this reminder it may need to be reset to be of any further use.

A more simple and functional type of alarm is the 'kitchen timer' type that generally consists of a simple clockwork mechanism that needs to be set in advance and then sounds a suitable audible note after the set amount of time has elapsed. These are very useful indeed as they are simple to carry around, lightweight and so cheap to buy that you can have several positioned around the house at very little cost. The only thing to remember is to make sure you react at the sound of the alarm. It is not much use setting an alarm and then ignoring the sound.

Use an alarm of this nature:

- To remind you to take medication.
- To remind you of stages in cooking (for example, when you need to turn the oven on).
- To remind you to get ready to go out at a set time.
- To remind you to go back to chores that need to be done in stages (having left items to soak, for example).
- To remind you if someone is coming to visit at a certain time.
- To remind you of a radio or TV programme you would like to watch.

Some wrist watches can also be programmed to be used as an alarm. If you are familiar with using a wrist watch as an alarm, it is a good thing to continue to do this. In any case, many people use their wrist watch to remind them of the date as well as time of day. But remember the advice above – if you are not used to using a wrist watch alarm, it is better to stick with a method you know and are familiar with.

When deciding what alarm method to use, remember the general rule quoted above: *do not try to learn something new to help your memory.* Use an alarm system you know and understand and that you find easy to manage. It doesn't matter how 'old fashioned' it may be; if it works for you, use it.

Laptops, tablets and mobile phones

If you are used to and happy to use a mobile phone, it can be very useful. It often has multiple functions including a diary and calendar and an alarm clock and reminder system. Some people use their mobile phone for all these functions and also to check emails, send short messages to friends and look up travel routes. To be honest, a mobile phone can be quite clumsy to use for some of these functions, but it does have the benefit of being small and light to carry and (by nature of this versatility) of eliminating the need for a diary, laptop, map and alarm clock. Most mobile phones also contain a camera that can be extremely useful.

Most older people, whilst quite happy to use a mobile phone for speaking to others on the move and perhaps for texting others and taking occasional photographs, do not make use of all its functions. If you need to be reminded of the time for regular events – taking medication, for example – then programming your mobile phone to remind you can be of great benefit if you are familiar with your phone and happy to use it.

Use a mobile phone, if you are happy with this method:

- To remind you of upcoming events and engagements.
- To remind you of meetings.
- To remind you that your car park ticket is running out.

Tablets and laptops also often incorporate an alarm, and if you are familiar with this kind of technology, then use the built-in alarm system to help your memory.

Self-set reminders (leaving something out)

This sounds like an odd method of memory jogging, but it often works. Say you have to take some items with you when you are due to leave the house. Leave those items on the floor immediately in front of the door by which you will leave the house. You will then definitely remember them.

In the same way:

- If you need to leave a cleaning product on for a certain amount of time before rinsing or flushing, leave an object out where you will see it and be reminded of the task.
- If you need to get the laundry off the line before leaving the house, leave a curtain half-closed so that your eye will be drawn to the window and remind you.
- If you need to add an ingredient to a dish half-way through cooking time, leave the ingredient near to the stove (as well as setting an alarm). This also works if you have to start cooking different dishes at different times – for example, if you need to cook vegetables to go with a main dish.
- If you need to take medication before a meal, put the dose on the table by your place setting.
- If you need to remember to post something – a birthday card, for example – leave it next to your house keys or handbag or whatever you take with you when you leave the house.

Lists

Lists are marvellous memory aids. They need no special equipment, as a simple pencil and paper work as well as anything. They are simple to make and simple to use. They focus the mind. They can act as a reminder of what you have done as well as what you have to do.

Use a list for:

- Shopping reminders.
- Household tasks that need to be done on a certain day.
- To remind you of calls you need to make or notes you need to write.
- To nudge your memory about upcoming events – such as gifts you need to buy, clothes you need to have washed and ironed, bags you need to pack.
- To remind you if a visitor is expected and you need to be prepared for them.

You may like to keep several lists for different tasks, but the most useful idea, especially if you have MCI, is to just keep one 'To do' list in a prominent place and remember to tick off items as you do them. You might like to have a separate page for each day and at the end of the day transfer over to the next day things you have not managed to complete.

The most important point to remember is that the list is supposed to be there to help you. Do not let it become your task master so that you get stressed if you have not completed your list. And do not become so obsessed by your 'To do' list that you cannot relax and enjoy your life. It can help to give each item on the list a 'star rating'; for example, three-star tasks are urgent but tasks with only one star can safely be left until tomorrow if you run out of time. Only do this if you do not find it too complicated to remember.

Example of a list

- Book dentist appointment *** (needs to be done today).
- Buy cat food * (not urgent – we still have enough for a couple of days).
- Buy birthday present for daughter ** (before end of week, when she is due to visit).

Other people

If your memory is not so good, one of the best supports you can have is another person. If your spouse or partner, your son or daughter or friend have a better memory than you, ask them to help. They might be very willing to help you to set an alarm, complete a 'To do' list, fill in your calendar or diary or even to telephone or text to remind you of things you need to do.

Just one proviso here: if you ask someone to help you in this way, do not be annoyed when they *do* give reminders! If you constantly say 'I knew that' when reminded, then your human reminder may decide not to bother. Remember that if you ask someone to help you by giving reminders, a 'thank you' for their help is most important. It can be irritating to be reminded but if you have asked someone else to help you, be glad when they do.

Names and faces

Most people who are worried about their memory will say that their biggest problem is with remembering the names of people and putting names to faces. There is a good reason for this. Names are actually quite random pieces of information. Many of our memories are linked to other memories of perhaps a certain time or event, and this helps us to recall them. Names do not generally have any 'linked' information. You may well remember someone's face and know perfectly well that you have met them before and even where you met them, but calling their name to mind can be difficult. There are several things you can do to help this.

- First, when you meet someone new, make sure that you hear their name clearly. Ask again if you do not hear it clearly the first time.
- Repeat the name after the introduction and try to say it several times in the conversation that follows (for example, 'So, Adam, did you have to come far today?' and 'How long have you known our host, Adam?').
- If you have time, try to link something about the face of the person you meet to their name. This is not always easy, but as an example, if you meet someone called 'Joan' and you have a daughter called Joan, it can help you to remember them the next time.

- When you say goodbye repeat the person's name again (for example, 'Goodbye, Adam. So nice to have met you').
- Tell people that your memory for names is not good and apologize in advance in case you forget.
- Don't be afraid to say something like 'It is silly of me, but although I know your face, I cannot remember your name'. (They may not remember yours either! So you can add 'I am Sally, by the way'.)
- If you have a partner, spouse or companion with you, ask them to remind you of the name of anyone you are going to meet beforehand.

Medicines

It is usually important to take medicines at certain times of the day and as frequently as your doctor tells you to take them. Some medicines work best before or after food and some have to be taken at regular intervals in order to work properly. It is therefore important to find a way to remember to take medicines when we should. There are many ways to remember, and we have mentioned some above:

- Set an alarm to remind you.
- Leave the medicine out where you will remember to take it; for example, if you have to take a pill at mealtimes, put the medicine bottle on the table where you eat. If you need to take it first thing in the morning, put it on the table by your bed.
- Add 'Take medicine' to your daily reminder list.

- Put 'Take medicine' on your calendar and tick it off when you have taken it.
- Programme your mobile phone to give you a reminder.
- Ask someone who lives with you to remind you.

If you have a condition that needs medication to be taken very regularly (such as diabetes or Parkinson's), it is very important that you take the trouble to make sure your reminder really works. If you are not sure that you will remember and the medication is very important, ask someone else to remind you.

It can be very dangerous to take too much of some medicines – an overdose. So, another sensible thing to do is to note when you have taken your medicine. You can ask for your pills to be given to you in a 'dosette' package. In this case each dose is placed in a foil container labelled with the day and time it needs to be taken. You can easily check if you have taken the dose because the container for that day and time will be empty if you have. This is a very good form of reminder if you are forgetful and if you live alone because you only have to check the packet to see if you have taken your medicine.

If you have a memory problem, then when your doctor prescribes medicine, always check how important it is to take the dose regularly. If you think you will easily forget your medicine, ask if you can be prescribed a different dose (for example, a once-a-day tablet instead of three times a day), or whether the medicine is really important to take.

As some medicines are very important, this is another area where you should not get angry or upset if someone living with you tries to help by reminding you to take your medication on time. Reminders like this mean that someone cares about you and wishes you well.

Spatial and route finders

'Spatial awareness' means being aware of where you are in relation to other things or other people. It is easy to become confused, especially in a strange place, and to take the wrong path or turn in the wrong direction. If you do this you may become lost and panic because you do not know where you are. There are things you can do to prevent or correct this.

To prevent yourself getting lost and confused:

- Take your time in a strange place – even if this means you move slowly and others get impatient with you.
- Pause occasionally to orientate yourself.
- Make a mental note of which turning you take or which door you go into.
- When you come out of a room in a strange place ask others which way to go to leave the building.

If you find you are lost:

- *Stop* and look around slowly. *Do not panic* and *do not carry on walking.*
- Breathe slowly and calmly. Retrace your steps if you can.

- Look around and see if you recognize any buildings, paths or roads.
- Do not be afraid to ask the way from a passer-by – you may have just missed the path.
- If you are really lost and have a mobile phone, call someone you know and ask them to help.

Finding your way

There are many new methods of route finding. Younger people often use their mobile phone as a kind of 'sat nav' and never consult a map at all. If you are confident with this kind of technology, then by all means use it. If you are not and if you are going to an unfamiliar place, try one of the following:

- Look at a map before you leave home.
- Note down the names of the roads you have to take to get to your destination.
- Draw a simple route map or ask someone to draw it for you.
- If you are driving, use a sat nav to help you.
- Take someone with you who will be your guide.

Equipment instructions

When you buy new items of equipment such as household appliances like washing machines or vacuum cleaners, they come with an instruction manual. Unfortunately, because these days the instructions have to be clear to everyone, you may find that they are written in several languages and that you have to wade your way through several pages before you find the one you can understand.

Sometimes instructions are shown as pictures (a hand pointing to a dial) rather than in words. You may find this helps but if you are used to following a series of written instructions, you may instead find this makes life more difficult.

Some electronic items like mobile phones and iPads do not have written instructions; instead the manufacturers expect you to 'download' their instruction book or to use their online system.

All of this may be very difficult for you if you have MCI. The simplest thing is to ask someone else to show you how to work the new appliance and to take the trouble to make sure you can do whatever you need to. It is also useful to ask someone you know to write the instructions down in a simple way for you. For example, if you have a new washing machine, it is likely that most of the time you will only need to use one or two programmes. Ask someone to write down a simple list of directions for those one or two programmes only, and stick the list up near the machine so that you can follow it every time you use it. It is a good idea to use a new piece of equipment as frequently as possible at first, as this will mean that your brain absorbs the pattern of the directions you use more easily.

If you are buying a new piece of household equipment, try to buy a model that is similar to whatever you had before so that you will find it easier to get used to.

Mobile phones

If you are using a new mobile phone, decide what functions you need the most. For example, with a phone you may just want to call and text others, perhaps. In that case, ask someone to coach you to use those functions and ignore any other functions until you need them. The assistants in mobile phone shops are usually very good at helping people to use their different phones and are used to older people needing some help, so you could go into a shop and ask them to train you.

If you only want to phone or text others, you could buy a simple phone that has these functions alone. This will make life easier for you. It is now possible to buy phones with larger-than-normal keypads for use by those with rheumatic fingers or people with poor eyesight. You can also get phones that allow you to programme your most common contacts to a one-touch button. Another useful function on some simple phones is a 'panic' button (usually on the reverse), which, if pressed, will contact someone close to you who can help you.

Remote controls

It is not just TVs that come with a remote control these days. Sound systems, room fans, electric fires and many other pieces of equipment now incorporate a remote control. This can be very confusing indeed, as all these remote controls look alike and mostly resemble modern landline telephones! There are many stories of people using their telephone to try to operate the TV or trying to dial a number on the TV remote, mistaking it for a telephone.

How can you deal with this problem? First, if you do not need to use a remote control for your equipment, then do not use it. Use the switches and controls on the equipment itself. This is, in many cases, easier to see and it prevents you being a 'couch potato' and avoiding moving from your comfy chair.

Where you do use a remote control, make an effort to learn the functions you will use most (for example, changing the channel on the TV) and leave the other functions alone. Label each remote control in large, easily read letters either by sticking on a label or by using a permanent marker pen on the casing itself. Before you use the control, check the label!

Always keep the remote controls in the same place and preferably have a different place for each one. This will help your brain to unconsciously recognize what you are using by associating it with the place in which it is kept.

Mnemonics and self-reminders

Mnemonics is a system such as a pattern of letters, ideas or associations that assist in remembering something. Some of us will recall being taught mnemonics such as 'Every Good Boy Deserves Fruit' to remember the names of musical notes or 'Richard of York Gave Battle In Vain' to remember the colours of the rainbow when we were at school. This is a very good system of remembering anything that has a sequence (like musical notes or colours of the rainbow), and you can make up your own to remember important lists. However, this kind of mnemonic needs to be easy to recall, otherwise you will spend hours trying to remember the mnemonic and it will rule you instead of helping you.

There are other very simple memory aids you may find work for you. One of my clients told me that if she went upstairs to fetch something, she named the item as she trod on each stair – 'library book, library book, library book', for example – and this worked very well for her in this case. Repetition can work well to help memory but it has its limitations. If you just repeat something two or three times and then dismiss it, the item is only committed to short-term memory and will quickly be lost. To be sure of recall you would need to keep repeating the item at intervals periodically.

Another way to commit things to memory is to make a picture in your mind – the sillier the better. Suppose you need to peel the potatoes, feed the dog and get the washing off the line before going out. Make a picture in your mind of potatoes hanging on the washing line and the dog trying to jump up to eat them.

Some people find that using their fingers as a memory aid can help. In the above case you would touch your thumb to note peeling the potatoes, your index finger to note feeding the dog and your middle finger to note taking in the washing. Then to recall each item you would touch the thumb and fingers.

Whichever form of memory aid you find useful, use it. Do not feel that you need to use a method someone else suggests, and do not feel silly for using such a method. If it works for you, it is a good method and it will help you to retain independence and to feel more confident.

The effect of tiredness and stress

If you are tired or under stress, any memory problems or confusion will get worse. It is worth keeping this in mind if you find yourself making a lot of mistakes or becoming confused. If you are tired, take a rest or go to bed early and you will almost certainly find that your memory and confusion will be much better after a rest or in the morning.

Think back to when you were at school and how stressful it could be when the teacher announced that you were having a test. Sometimes every fact you knew seemed to fly out of the window as soon as you thought you were going to be tested. It can be like that if someone suddenly asks you for your phone number – the mind can become a complete blank. When you are put 'on the spot' your brain sometimes seems to freeze.

There are some things you can do to help:

- Save difficult or complicated tasks for a time when you are feeling fresh. Don't attempt to do them when you are tired or under pressure.
- Step back from a difficult situation and try a relaxing few breaths. You could say 'I need a minute to think' or just make an excuse, 'I'm in a hurry now – I'll need to come back later'.

- Don't put yourself under more pressure by desperately trying to think of something you have forgotten. It is better to put it out of your mind and the answer will probably pop into your brain as soon as you relax.
- Keep a note of your address and phone number in your purse or wallet so you can look them up easily.
- If someone is with you, ask them to help. Don't be upset – everyone has blank moments.
- In general, try not to become overtired or have too many tasks lined up. Remember the advice given under 'lists' and leave what is not urgent until tomorrow or the day after.

Tiredness and stress affect everyone. The only difference is that younger people can sometimes overcome the fatigue and the worry and perform when they have to, even though they are tired or stressed. Older people find this more difficult. It isn't important. If you are older, you are also hopefully wiser. You understand that you need to give yourself time and space. Take your time and give yourself the space.

The term 'mild cognitive impairment' means that your cognition (your ability to remember and to function every day) is impaired (faulty), but *only mildly*. You are still able to help yourself to function better and to manage your activities of daily living (ADLs) so that you can manage to live independently.

Using memory aids – of whatever kind – to help you to function and live independently is both sensible and wise.

Do not feel that by using memory aids you are failing or giving way. If you had a broken leg you would be happy to use a crutch until the leg mended. Memory aids are the 'crutch' for cognitive impairment. Use them and keep your independence.

Key points

- Using aids to help you remember something is not a weakness; it is sensible and helps you to be independent.
- Diaries and calendars in whatever form suits you are a basic standby to jog memory.
- Alarms come in many forms and they are very useful. Use the ones that suit you best.
- Do not try to learn a new form of technology or learning to help you remember. It is better to use a tried and trusted system you are familiar with.
- The timing of some medication is important: make every effort to take your medicine on time.
- If you find it easy to lose your way, use memory aids to help or to ask for help from other people.
- Take the time to learn how to use new equipment or aids. If you don't need to learn all the functions, just learn the ones you will use.
- Don't try to learn new things if you are tired or stressed.
- Don't be upset if your memory gets worse when you are tired or stressed.

Chapter 7

Thinking about the Future

Most people do some limited planning for the future. We are all generally familiar with the idea of thinking about careers, family, pensions and property in terms of planning for the years ahead. Far-sighted people will have made plans for their retirement, considering both the financial and social aspects.

It is interesting, if you ask anyone in mid-life about their plans for their future, that generally even forward-thinking people have only considered a future where they have family within reach and where they have all their 'faculties' to enjoy retirement. Very few people consider the possibility that they may become frail, that their family may move far away, or that they may develop cognitive problems and need intensive support.

No one wants to consider such a future, and this is probably why very few people make provision for it. If you are reading this book, then very probably you are beyond 'middle age' and any plans you make may be more immediate. If you have been told that you (or perhaps your life-partner) have mild cognitive impairment (MCI), this can act as a wake-up call and you will find that you have to consider your future plans in a hurry.

This chapter looks at some of the things you should consider (others are discussed in Chapter 2), and how you can plan ahead so that problems concerning health, finances and residential matters can be managed in the best way for you.

Planning finances

Money and finance is an area where many people do plan ahead. Government policy on pensions in the UK has meant that even those who previously assumed that the State would provide for their old age have been forced to think in a more personal vein.

This book is not meant to reiterate advice that can be obtained through other means. Financial advice about planning for the future can easily be obtained, even for those who have very limited means, and some sources of advice are given in Chapter 10, in the list of support organizations at the end of the book.

In this chapter we take a different look at the financial side of getting old and try to consider just what we might really want in the way of material things in the future. If you talk to younger people just starting out on life, they are likely to be considering saving into a pension fund for their later years. At this stage of life most people considering the future acknowledge that the responsibility to arrange a pension fund is important. In later middle age, too, people often think and plan to ensure that their retirement will be comfortable and that they will be able to afford the material things they think they will need.

Rather strangely, in later life, when those who made these sensible plans and arrangements so that they would be able to pay for any extra aids or assistance they might need are actually required to use the money saved for that purpose, they may be reluctant to do so. The most common reason given for not using capital or savings to help oneself is the wish to leave a legacy for children or grandchildren.

This book is not the place to discuss whether accepting state aid (which, after all, is simply money paid by other people) is morally right or wrong. However, it is pertinent for anyone in the position where they finally need to use money set aside for 'old age' to stand back and ask why they might choose to lead less comfortable lives in order to give their children or grandchildren a legacy.

One of the biggest difficulties of financial planning for the future is that we generally don't know what the length of that future is to be. None of us know how long we are likely to live, and except in very rare cases, we cannot anticipate how much of our future life might be a time of high dependency (which generally means high expense) or how much of this time might come under the control of others, such as younger family members or those to whom we grant power of attorney (POA).

In Chapter 2 we considered the action of granting POA and looked closely at choosing who you might appoint as your attorney. Although this seems a major step to some, others regard it as a simple and sensible action, 'just in case'.

Probably the most important thing to remember is that granting POA to someone is not an irrevocable step. Even once it is registered, you can rescind it and make another one, provided you still have the capacity to do so. Knowing this fact may make you more likely to consider taking action to draw up a POA so that others can help you to manage your finances, if need be.

Other matters concerning a financial future are more difficult to plan for. Everyone seems to know these days that residential care in a 'care home' is very expensive. Indeed, one of the reasons people avoid this option as long as possible is because care home fees eat into savings at an alarming rate. There are financial plans that act as a kind of 'insurance'[1] against the possibility of a need for care home fees. Usually you pay a lump sum up front that will cover any fees that may arise, and the gamble is whether care home fees that need to be paid will be more than the lump sum paid.

Many people worry that their home will have to be sold to fund their place in a residential care home. This is probably the most common concern. Some people try to arrange a legal 'trust' to ensure that their home will not have to be sold to cover care home fees. This can be a sensible arrangement, but it is important to find out the legal position first. At present your home will not be considered when contributions to care home fees are calculated if a family member who is aged over 60 lives there.

You may, of course, be gambling on the notion that you will never need residential care.

Planning for support

Financial planning for the future is usually acknowledged to be a good idea, but what many people do not consider is the possibility – even the likelihood – that they will need support of a different kind in their later years. Think about this now. The likelihood is that you may need help and support for activities of everyday living. You may need help with transport, shopping, gardening or housework.

There are many reasons why this possibility is not planned for. The most common reason is simply that no one likes to think that the time will come when they will be frail or disabled and need either physical help or support for their everyday activities of living.

When most people think about their retirement they see themselves freed from the 'slavery' of earning a wage – living a more relaxed lifestyle, enjoying the time and opportunity to take up new hobbies, enjoy cultural pursuits, travelling and seeing more of their wider family. These future visions tend to encompass things like cruises, University of the Third Age (U3A), visiting local attractions, giving more time to a hobby such as golf or supporting the local football team and perhaps volunteering or helping to care for grandchildren. People look forward to being able to have a lie-in, see more films or shows, tend to the garden, visit the local pub, or having time to take up a new hobby.

Few people spend time contemplating losing their driving licence because of disability, experiencing increasing problems with mobility, losing their sight or hearing, death of a long-term partner, serious illness, constant hospital appointments, difficulty with cooking or shopping or any of the myriad other problems that can, in many cases, dog the days of seniors and make later years a constant worry.

How easy is it to calculate whether you will need support to manage your everyday life in five years? ...in ten years? ...in twenty years? No one wants to become morbid or fixated on unfortunate things that *might* happen, but it can be worthwhile sometimes to give a little thought to the 'what ifs' of life:

- Suppose you have to give up your driving licence due to poor sight or other health problems; do you know if there are any bus or train services, where the bus stops are, which bus routes you might want to use and what other forms of transport are available to you? Could you get to your doctors' surgery or to the supermarket easily?
- Suppose your spouse or partner dies suddenly; would you want to live alone in your present accommodation? Could you manage this? Where would you choose to move to if not? Could you afford to move? Could you manage to live alone?
- If you (or a partner) became ill or disabled, do you know where the hospital is and how to reach it? What are the waiting times like for operations? When are the visiting hours?
- If you or a partner were no longer able to cook, how would you manage? Are there any local community meals services (Meals on Wheels)? What do ready meals taste like and where can you get them? Are there any good local eating places?

- If your mobility becomes a problem, how would you manage shopping? Is there a local taxi service? Do your local stores deliver? Would you have to make orders online and do you know how? Is there someone who could help you?

Moving home

Moving house is a big step, especially if you are planning to leave a house where you have brought up a family and where you have perhaps lived for many years. Even if logically you know that having a smaller, more easily run house (perhaps nearer to your children or other family members) makes sense, it can still be a severe wrench to move away from the people you know, the shops you are used to, the clubs or groups you have become accustomed to, and all the 'networks' you may have formed over a long period.

Interestingly, adult children are often the biggest proponents of such a move. It can be quite a shock to suddenly realize that the children you have nurtured, protected and guided for years are now trying to protect and guide *you*. But so often this is the case and equally often children are at the forefront of suggesting a move that brings you nearer to where they live.

What causes people to move house in later life? Perhaps it is the sensible and mature thought and planning that is part of your overall retirement plan.

Or perhaps it is the result of a health crisis that convinces you that you need a house that is smaller, more easily run and nearer to those who will be able to offer you support.

Sometimes it is the death of a partner or a spouse that brings an inherent loneliness to the fore and a realization that you would like to be near your remaining family.

Sometimes there are financial reasons why 'downsizing' is a good idea.

Whatever the reason, a house move in later life can be a major shock and upset in your life. Even if you are pleased about the move, have been desiring it for a while, and find the perfect new home to move into, the change can be disruptive and unsettling.

I often have first contact with clients who have recently moved house. Some minor memory or cognitive problems that have been experienced but that have been managed (or perhaps ignored) in a familiar scenario may often come to the fore after a house move and a diagnosis of dementia may follow. It is unlikely that the house move has 'caused' the dementia – as we have seen in previous chapters, dementia takes many years to develop. But the change to familiar routines, the need to learn new routes to local places and the requirement to form new networks (doctors, dentists, shops, libraries and public transport arrangements) can all exacerbate the beginnings of cognitive decline.

One of the first problems people with dementia encounter is a difficulty in learning anything new. To a certain extent this occurs in all of us as we age, but those whose cognition is intact will only find learning new networks more difficult, whilst those with dementia may find it impossible.

It may seem as though I am suggesting that moving house is a bad thing. Of course, I am not suggesting this. Very often moving home to somewhere smaller, more easily run, nearer to amenities and closer to your family is the best decision you can take. What I have shown, however, is that a house move late in life, or when already cognitively challenged, can make memory difficulties seem much worse.

Suppose you have decided to move home for any of a number of good and sensible reasons. Is there anything you can do that will help to mitigate the possibility that your cognition will suffer? I believe there are many things that you and those around you can do to help.

I have explained elsewhere[2] the manner in which our brain learns new skills and routines and how some skills (like driving a car) become 'hard-wired' into the brain so that we can carry out actions without consciously thinking about them. In a similar way, we become used to routes in our locality. If we are walking to the local shops for the paper and if this is an action we carry out every day, then we do not have to consciously plan out our route or consider what we will do when we reach the shop. It is most likely that we walk to the shop whilst thinking about something else and that when we reach the shop, we walk in, pick up our 'usual' paper, and pay for it with barely a thought. This inherent knowledge of your home locality and the routines you have become used to are now part your life.

My first suggestion, then, is that you become knowledgeable about the new area into which you are going to move. If you are moving nearer to family, it is likely that you will have stayed in the new area before and will have had a chance to learn about it. This is an excellent start, but you can take it further. When staying with family or friends we tend to be guided by them as to where we go and what we do. But when you move, the new area is to become *your* neighbourhood, so the paths you take and the shops you frequent may not be the ones your family or friends use.

Take some time to look around the area. In this respect, technology can be a great help. These days you do not have to actually visit an area to see what it looks like. Use technology (such as Google Maps) to have a 'virtual' look around the area. It can be fascinating to do your exploring in this way, and once you become familiar with the technology, you will find it is really useful. You can 'walk' or 'drive' along a route, peer round corners, view a shopping centre from the air, see how near the local parks are to your home, and all without leaving your own screen.

If computers are not your thing, you can still make use of other forms of information. There are excellent photographs, films, books and tourist leaflets that can be obtained through your local library so that you can become familiar with your new locality. Of course, visits to the area are the best thing, and a few weekends or days spent exploring the new locality, even before you move there, will pay dividends in terms of becoming familiar with the area.

Do not just focus on your family if you are planning to move closer to them. They will be an important part of your new life and routine, but not the whole of it. Find out about local clubs and organizations you might be interested in.

If you are down on a visit, see if you can attend club meetings as a visitor. Usually tourist boards have lists of clubs and local organizations, or these days you can 'search the web' to see what goes on in the area. Don't forget local libraries, as these are often a prime source of information.

Find out about as many local shops as possible and sources of services like car servicing, household appliance repairs, hair stylists, gyms and exercise clubs (if this interests you) as well as local amenities like parks and nature reserves, household waste disposal (the tip), libraries and education centres. Naturally, part of the fun of moving to a new area involves exploring and finding out where things are and deciding for yourself which shops to patronize and where the best pub is for Sunday lunch. I am not suggesting that you make all your lifestyle decisions before you move home, but knowing a bit more about the choice available makes life more interesting and less overwhelming at first.

I suggest that when it comes to the actual practicalities and management of the move, you accept any offer to help or make things easier. Most removal firms nowadays offer a packing service, so why not take advantage of this when you are moving later in life. Perhaps plan your move so that you do not move out of one house and into another all on the same day. Many firms will store your furniture for a day or two so that you can arrange to have the new house cleaned before you move in, perhaps, or make sure any vital repairs or renovations are done. If you are moving nearer to children or other family, they might let you stay for a short whilst until your new home is ready for occupation.

If you have any cognitive problems, take a lot of time to become familiar with the new area. Walk or drive any routes you will use frequently with a friend, partner or family member until you feel totally confident about finding your way. Examine local maps so that you can find out about any shortcuts. Think ahead about alternative routes in case of roadworks or diversions. It might be helpful to ask your new neighbours the best way to go.

It is very important not to focus wholly on any family or friends who are already living in the area. You will need to forge your own networks if you are to feel relaxed and familiar with the area and not become a burden to your family and friends. If you already have a hobby or belong to an organization that is networked throughout the country – for example, charities such as Rotary clubs or political parties – you will be able to ask for an introduction to your new local branch or club. This can be helpful, although it is important to remember that even clubs that have the same aim are populated with different people and they may have a different atmosphere to the one you are used to. Try to keep an open mind and become familiar with the locals before you decide that the new club is not for you.

If you do find yourself getting lost or becoming confused after a house move, do not panic and assume that you have finally 'lost it'. Older people will always take longer to settle into any new routine or learn new routes and get to know people. Remember that you can afford to take your time. Most probably you are no longer working and so there is not the same pressure to get to places on time or to fit jobs into a small time slot. One idea is to allow yourself double the time you normally would to get to any new place or to carry out any new routine. Once you feel under less pressure you are more likely to relax and find it easy to remember what to do and where to go.

In short, it is more difficult for older people (and especially those who have MCI) to learn a new routine or become accustomed to a new place and to new people. But 'more difficult' does not mean 'impossible'. Allow more time to do things or get to places, consider carefully how you are going to go about arranging an outing or making an appointment, and expect to have to repeat things more often before they become familiar. You will get there in the end.

Residential care or nursing homes

Perhaps you have made your family 'promise' never to place you in a residential care home. How sure are you that your family will be able to keep such a promise?

Most of us do not want to contemplate having to live in a residential care home at the end of our lives, and yet for many people, this is the reality. There are good reasons why living in a residential care home may be the best option at some stage in our lives, but the most common reason is a disability of some kind – either a physical or cognitive disability.

The cost of residential care makes most people try every alternative first, and the notion that our children may want to 'put us away' is probably a false one. It is worth taking a few minutes to contemplate the notion of residential care in a care or nursing home, to be sure of your reasons for rejecting the idea – as indeed most people do reject it. What is it about it that upsets people so much?

- Many people cite the *loss of independence* as the reason for refusing residential care. When considering this idea, it is worth remembering that care homes or nursing homes are not prisons. I remember being very surprised when a client of mine said she did not want her mother to move to a care home because she enjoyed her outings so much. When I pointed out that she could still have outings when living in the residential home, the daughter said that she thought that once you had entered a residential care home you were not allowed to leave it. Possibly the fact that residential homes these days generally have doors unlocked via an electronic keypad may be the reason for this misconception.

  A residential care or nursing home is meant to be a home, not a prison. All residents (except in unusual circumstances) are there of their own free will and are at liberty to come and go as they would in their own home. True, most residents will only leave the home accompanied by a friend or relative, but this is usually because they are frail, disabled or confused, and need a companion to help them.

  As for other forms of independence, if you are capable of washing, dressing and attending to your own personal care, the staff will be only too glad to leave you to do this. The truth is that most people choose residential care because they are unable to manage these things themselves and actually need the help that is offered.

- Another objection commonly raised is the notion of *having to live a communal life*. Many people object to living so closely with a number of other people. It is true that in a residential home, meals are served at set times and there will generally be activities that are organized to happen on certain days. However, no one is forced to take part in activities, and these days good homes always offer alternatives to set meal times, for example, snacks served in your room. Residents are encouraged to mix with others, but this is not compulsory.

After doing some careful thinking you may still be of the strong opinion that you do not ever want to accept residential or nursing home care. Alternatively, you may now have come to the conclusion that this type of care is the best option in certain circumstances.

Whichever of these two conclusions you reach, the possibility is that you will, like it or not, at some stage in your life need to live in a residential or nursing home (perhaps only for a short time, such as for convalescence after a hospital stay).

If this is a strong possibility, it is a good idea to think in advance about:

- What sort of home you would prefer?
- What aspects of your life and routine are really important to you?

- Making decisions about these two criteria.
- Writing down your wishes so that your carers and family can know your wishes if you are unable to tell them.

What sort of home would you prefer?

Residential care homes can be small and 'family-run', or large and organized. Some homes are modern and purpose-built; others are in houses or buildings that have been adapted for use. Older buildings generally have more 'character' and seem more interesting, but purpose-built homes are usually easier to get around, and are laid out in a well-thought-out manner.

Homes may have extensive gardens or smaller outside space. Most have some kind of exterior space, but if you are fond of gardens, you may want to choose a home with pleasant open grounds. Some homes have a big programme of outings and activities; others are more centred round the internal community. Some people love lots of outings and events; others feel safer in a quieter, more homely and inward-looking place.

There are homes with large communal areas; others are built around small 'units' of six to eight residents, to create a 'family' atmosphere. Some homes are in quite remote areas where it is peaceful and quiet; others are built in areas where residents can watch the busy community going by each day.

Often the decision to choose residential or nursing care is not made by the person to be cared for, but by their carers and family. Are you sure that your family know what is really important to you? For example:

- Do you like a cooked breakfast, or do you prefer cereal and toast, or no breakfast at all?
- Do you like to have quiet times without background music or the TV?
- Do you like to be able to step outside for fresh air whenever you choose?
- Do you like a drink before dinner or after dinner?
- Do you hate being alone without company?
- Do you hate being in a crowded room with a TV permanently switched on?
- Do you like to stay up late or get up early?

These may not be the important areas of your life or routine that are important to *you*, but this list gives you an idea of what to consider if you are contemplating residential care. The truth is that because so few people give any consideration to the possibility of needing residential care in the future, very few people end up living in the kind of residential care home they would like.

By thinking about this in advance and making your wishes known to your families, you increase the possibility that if 'the worst happens', at least it is likely to be on terms that you like and can accept.

Accepting help

No one wants to feel that they are a 'burden' to others. We would all like to manage our own lives adequately and many people really hate asking for help. Why is this?

One reason people don't ask for help is because they do not want to feel beholden to others. As we age we tend to feel that younger members of the family or of the community around us are managing better than we are, and we do not want to feel under an obligation to busy people.

However, it is often true that simply because you are older and perhaps less mobile you may be in a position to easily return favours. A younger neighbour may happily help you out by collecting some shopping and in return you can take in deliveries for them. Or perhaps you could walk their dog whilst they are at work and they in return might mow your lawn occasionally. If you are a grandparent you can often be useful in a childminding capacity and not feel under an obligation if you need to ask your children to give you a lift to appointments.

Frequently my older clients tell me that they don't want to worry their adult children or ask for help because their offspring are 'so busy'. On the other hand, when a crisis happens, the adult children will say to me, 'Why didn't my mum ask me for help? I would have been happy to be there rather than have this [crisis] happen.' If you have elderly parents, do not just blithely assume that they are 'managing' because they do not ask for help. Keep your eyes open when you visit and make your offers of support tactfully.

There is food for thought there.

It is also worth remembering that people often actually like helping others. The biggest difficulty for those willing to help is knowing what is needed. When my husband was ill, my next-door neighbour was delighted when I asked her to pick up some shopping for me. 'I've been wanting to offer you some help', she said, 'but I didn't know what you needed and I thought you might be offended if I just turned up.' I soon put her at ease in that respect.

Another elderly client told me that she would really like it if her poorly neighbour in the flat upstairs asked her to do an errand. 'I don't like to knock on the door in case she is asleep. I know she is not very well and I would hate to be the one who wakes her up.' Eventually she agreed with this neighbour that any help required could be requested by a note through the letterbox.

If you are in need of help, it is worth thinking carefully about where you can get that help. It is also important to be up-front and ask for exactly what you want. For example, 'Please could you pick up my prescription for me on your way home from work?' is a good way of framing a request rather than, 'I just wondered if you had any time on your hands?'

In a similar way, if you would like to help a friend or neighbour, be clear about what you can and cannot do. 'Would you like me to sit with Fred whilst you go to your doctor's appointment?' or 'Shall I mow your front lawn whilst I've got the mower out?' is better than a vague, 'Let me know if I can do anything.'

If you do not want to ask others for 'favours' and if you can afford it, then help of many kinds can be had if you are prepared to pay.

Several volunteer organizations offer to drive people who have no transport to appointments, and these usually ask for a donation simply to cover petrol costs. Some local authorities offer a door-to-door bus service that is bookable in advance. Taxi services are usually able to cater for people who have limited mobility, and several will have lifts and wheelchair access. There are also specialist businesses that offer driver and companionship services in many areas.

Most doctors' surgeries and pharmacies now offer a prescription pick-up and home delivery service. There are many private cleaning and gardening services, so you can choose to have help for the jobs you can no longer manage whilst continuing to take care of everyday chores and light cleaning or gardening that you can handle.

Most people think of care agencies as supplying help with bathing and dressing for those who can no longer manage these daily tasks alone. Care agencies do, indeed, give this kind of help, but you may not know that they will also help to prepare meals, do light housework and even just provide company and companionship.

Accepting limited help when you need it can ensure that you do not need to make the bigger life-changing decisions – moving home, going into residential care – too soon or even at all. It is worth remembering this when you are refusing support or insisting that you 'can manage'.

Details of many of these services can be found listed in Chapter 10.

Key points

- When planning for the future, remember that you may need to think about disabilities and frailty as well as relaxation and retirement.
- Remember that money you have saved for your 'old age' is meant to be used to help you be independent.
- Moving home is a major step and may not always be the best option.
- If you do move home in later life, take the trouble to familiarize yourself with your new area and networks.
- There are many forms of support, and accepting help when we need it can avoid a crisis developing.
- Help can be given freely by friends and neighbours as well as family.
- Help and support can also be hired and paid for.
- Residential care may be unavoidable at some stage, so it is useful to consider your likes and dislikes.

Endnotes

1   See www.payingforcare.org
2   Jordan, M. (2014) *The Essential Carer's Guide to Dementia*. London: Hammersmith Health Books.

Chapter 8

Can Dementia Be Prevented after a 'Diagnosis' of MCI?

Most doctors will tell you that there is no such thing as a 'diagnosis' of mild cognitive impairment (MCI) because it is not a disease in itself. It is a term used to describe a situation where someone is aware (or those around them are aware) of memory and cognitive failings – a slowing down of abilities, a reduction in faculties, and more difficulties in managing everyday life than previously experienced. MCI is considered to involve problems with memory, problem-solving, language and judgement, but not to the extent that this prevents normal functioning. As a general rule, a person in this situation can still manage their activities of daily living (ADLs), and will not have a significantly low score when taking a 'memory test'.

As explained in Chapter 1, progress from MCI to dementia is not inevitable. Figures for the 'conversion rate' to dementia vary, according to different studies.[1]

It is thought by some that about half of those with MCI progress to dementia within three to five years. Some others do not progress to dementia, but their cognition does not improve before the end of their life. Some others are diagnosed and treated for other conditions which, when treated, resolve the MCI. Some people seem to 'spontaneously' improve and do not progress to dementia.

It is possible that people whose cognition improves get better because they pay attention to areas of their lifestyle that affect their brain health. This is an area of interest that is presently attracting a lot of attention in the media as well as from health professionals. There is still only very limited accredited research to indicate that it is possible to improve cognition by attention and alterations to lifestyle, but information about this possibility will be discussed in this chapter.

What happens to the brain in dementia?

Dementia is the name given to a collection of symptoms – chiefly, memory lapses, impaired intellectual function and difficulty in carrying out the functions of everyday life – which are caused by any of more than 200 diseases. Alzheimer's disease, for example, which people often think is just another word for dementia, is actually just one of the diseases that cause dementia symptoms.

Although a huge amount of research has been done, and although many theories have been put forward, the truth is that no one knows what causes dementia. It is currently thought that there may be multiple factors, some genetic, some relating to lifestyle, and some perhaps relating to inflammation or to trauma, either physical or mental.

We know that during dementia brain cells lose their ability to communicate with each other and that when this happens, they die. As more brain cells die, so inter-cell communication becomes even harder, causing a 'cascade' effect as more and more brain cells die. Whilst this is happening there is a build-up of some proteins in the brain. These form clumps (called plaques) and tangles. Different diseases (forms of dementia) involve different proteins and these become toxic, causing more harm to the remaining brain cells. As the brain cells are damaged or killed, the brain becomes less able to retrieve and rebuild memories, and people who have dementia become progressively less able to carry out different functions, to think and plan ahead and to solve problems. Eventually, as the disease progresses, even simple actions like eating and drinking cause problems, and people who have dementia are no longer able to live independently.

When does dementia start? In mid-life?

We know that people are more likely to develop dementia as they age (although sometimes quite young people can develop dementia, so age is not the only factor involved), and we also know that the symptoms of dementia only show after considerable damage has been done to the brain. As I explained in Chapter 1, I often liken what happens to the experience of driving around a town. If a road is closed (perhaps owing to road works), traffic will be diverted down a different route. Should you be taking this alternative route and find it congested due to, say, a traffic accident, you might turn off down a side road if you know the area and find your way to your destination by taking a series of diversions that do not constitute a direct route, but nevertheless get you where you plan to go. When areas of the brain are damaged, the thinking, planning and actioning process might need to take a longer route than the direct way, and the brain is very good at using such diversions to get where it needs to go. Mostly we are unaware of this 'diversion' process. However, there is a limit. I always explain that symptoms of dementia appear when the brain has run out of 'alternative routes'. It can no longer find its way, even using diversions.

Some doctors now believe that it can take up to 20 years for the brain to be so damaged that the symptoms of dementia begin to show. If this is true, dementia probably begins in mid-life, and the time to be thinking about avoiding dementia is not when you are 60 or 70 years old, but when you are 40 or so.

Why is dementia progressive and 'incurable'?

What do we mean when we say a disease is 'progressive'? One of my clients recently suggested that it would be better to call dementia a 'regressive' disease because people who have dementia appear to regress – they become less and less able to carry out everyday functions. We know that if you have a diagnosis of dementia it is almost certain that your symptoms will get worse over time – the symptoms will 'progress'.

At the moment, conventional medicine has no treatment that provides a cure for the symptoms of dementia and no drug that will stop its progress. People who have MCI do not have a diagnosis of dementia, and so there are some who think that if you have MCI, you have a 'window of opportunity' to take steps to prevent the development of dementia symptoms.

Conventional medical thinking

Practitioners of conventional medicine (that is, your doctor, consultant physician or consultant psychiatrist) are often asked by patients who have been told that they have MCI, what can be done about it and more importantly, perhaps, what can be done to prevent MCI developing into dementia? Indeed, when I have been present in the diagnostic clinic I have listened to various doctors struggling to find the right advice to give in these instances. They want to be helpful and kind, but the truth is that the conventional approach suggests that there is little to be done. This is because we do not know the ultimate cause of dementia.

Most often the doctor will give some general advice about eating a good diet and taking exercise along with suggestions that 'what is good for the heart is good for the brain' with reference to lifestyle. Most will also tell patients not to worry, that they should go away and enjoy life and 'go on as you are doing now'. I have heard this advice being given many times and sometimes patients are reassured by it but sometimes they have asked me later if there is really nothing that they can do to 'tip the odds' against dementia.

With the best will in the world, the most that doctors of conventional medicine can do is give this kind of reassurance and suggest that those who are worried return in a few months or sooner if they notice any further symptoms that worry them.

Conventional medical thinking is often very much concerned with early diagnosis, and if you read current research, this, too, lays great emphasis on early diagnosis.[2] However, dementia is one of the diseases where early diagnosis makes very little difference to the outcome. The most that can happen is that people with a diagnosis can then get valuable support and can be guided to make plans for the future, when symptoms will get worse.

As someone who has been used to providing support for people with dementia and their families, I have to say that support is very useful, and referral to a dementia adviser or dementia support worker (referred to as 'dementia supporters' from now on) is one of the positive things a doctor can do to help. There are two things that make this strategy less successful, however.

The first is that if people are referred soon after diagnosis and the dementia is still in the early stages, offers of support are frequently refused by the patient. This is because the symptoms are not too difficult to manage and many people, despite being informed that the disease is progressive, have no conception that what they are coping with easily now will become extremely difficult to manage later. I know that this does happen because of the large numbers of clients who have refused help initially but who contact me again after many months or even years.

The second factor that is unhelpful to those with MCI is that dementia supporters are specifically trained and employed to help people with dementia. If you have MCI, you are not considered to have dementia, and the help of the dementia supporter is not open to you.

This is one of the prime reasons I have for writing this book.

Some alternatives

So what could you do if you want to be proactive rather than the 'go away and enjoy life' suggestions you might get from your doctor?

Address health issues

At the very least you can do your best to address any health issues that are known to be associated with a higher risk of dementia. In this respect I would suggest that you pay particular attention to the following:

- *Type 2 diabetes (also known as 'maturity onset' diabetes)*: this is known to be a risk factor for dementia. Because diabetes is treatable these days, many people treat a diagnosis of diabetes as a minor inconvenience. But diabetes is a serious condition: it can result in problems with blood circulation that can affect the eyes, heart and peripheral parts of the body such as fingers and toes. It is known that people with MCI who also have diabetes are three times more likely to develop dementia than those who have only MCI.[3]

There is now ample evidence that changes in lifestyle can control and possibly even cure type 2 diabetes.[4] So, if you are diagnosed with type 2 diabetes, it is vital that you take control of the situation through diet and lifestyle changes and that you *do not* simply assume that medication and your health adviser will deal with the situation. This is one instance where the solution (and a possible development of dementia) is within your control.

- *Hearing loss*: there is a known association between hearing loss and dementia. Studies suggest that a hearing impediment is associated with a 30–40 per cent rate of accelerated cognitive decline.[5] You can read more about this in Chapter 3. Although the reasons for the association between hearing loss and dementia are still not completely clear, it is wise to take sensible precautions. As mentioned in Chapter 3, there is a supposition that for those hard of hearing the effort to hear diverts resources away from other cognitive functions. So, if you are a little deaf, do not strain to hear if you can improve the situation by moving to a quieter place, turning up the volume, turning off distracting background sound or using other senses (sight, touch) to help in understanding what is being said. Keep away from noisy environ-ments. If it has been suggested that you need a hearing aid, invest in the best you can afford.

Then take the trouble to get used to it so that it becomes an 'aid' and not a distraction. Persistence is very important here and there is more at stake than just being isolated from society. You should also make use of hearing loops, lip reading or subtitles. Pretending that you do not need help for hearing is not brave; it is foolhardy and opens you more to the risk of dementia.

- *Heart disease and stroke*: one form of dementia, called 'vascular dementia', which is the most common form of dementia after Alzheimer's disease, develops where problems with blood circulation result in parts of the brain not receiving enough blood and oxygen. This is known to be associated with some forms of heart disease[6] and with stroke, even tiny strokes (commonly known as transient ischaemic attacks or TIA). If you have been diagnosed with heart disease of any kind, then do not treat it lightly. Follow your doctor's advice. If you do not have a history of heart disease, follow a sensible lifestyle in order to avoid heart disease if possible. If you have previously had a stroke, bear in mind that recovery is possible and can continue for many months and even years following the initial stroke.
- *Falls*: take care of your eyesight and follow a sensible exercise programme to maintain your strength and balance. Falls can be a major cause of increasing frailty as we get older. In some areas special classes are available to help improve balance and fitness in the elderly. Take advantage of these if they are available.

Reduce stress in your life

Some stress is good for us. You should not feel that you have to remove all sources of stress from your life – this would make for a very dull existence. It is known that stress can contribute to ill health if it is caused by situations over which we have no control. So, if you find you are becoming stressed about something you can do nothing about, consider using a therapy such as meditation, yoga or mindfulness to change the way you view your life and to help you to cope.

If your stress is caused by the actions of someone else such as a family member and you cannot influence the cause of the stress (by talking to them or taking some action), consider counselling to help you deal with the way their actions affect you. It can be very hard to relinquish worrying about children or other loved ones, but think about whether your worry and the stress it causes you is actually doing anything to help the situation.

Holistic approaches

'Holistic' isn't another word for 'alternative'; it simply means 'whole body'; that is, a holistic approach is an approach to health that does not take symptoms in isolation but considers the whole body (and mind) when looking for a healthcare solution. In this case, we take the symptoms that indicate MCI and consider how these might be an indicator of something wrong in our general health. Few people – and very few doctors – have in the past taken a 'holistic approach' to cognitive problems because it is not generally recognized that any of a number of physical health problems can also have an effect on the brain and cognition.

Recently a few doctors and researchers have begun to consider a holistic approach,[7] and this is currently an area of interest, especially now that more research into greater numbers of cases with cognitive problems other than dementia is being published.

We do not yet know the cause of most types of dementia or the reasons why some people succumb to it and others do not. The same is true of many other diseases. We do not know what causes them or why some people get some diseases and others do not. A number of medical practitioners are beginning to rethink the way that medical treatment is approached now, and suggesting that rather than treat diseases when they occur, we should consider how best to bolster the health of the human body so that it is able to resist disease:[8]

> The problem with prion disorders is a similar problem to cancer. A pathological process has been switched on which has a momentum of its own – indeed I think of prion disorders as protein cancers. Stopping a smoker from smoking does not cure his lung cancer – it is too late...by the time the clinical picture arises it is too late for curative treatment.[9]

That may sound radical, but it makes a lot of sense.

It is now known, for example, that cells in our body are mutating all the time, and that if these mutating cells were left to proliferate, these mutations would lead to cancer.

The reason this does not happen is that the body generally 'recognizes' these aberrant cells and destroys them before they grow and become a cancerous growth. No one is quite sure yet why some cancerous cells escape the notice of the body's defence systems, but it is suggested that by strengthening body systems and maintaining optimum health, we can help the bodily defences perform their job better.

In the same way, no one is quite sure which of the many hypothesized 'triggers' may actually cause dementia. It is not even knows why some people with MCI develop dementia and others do not. At this stage of medical knowledge no one is even able to predict whether a particular person who has MCI will get worse or better or stay the same. But it may be that by strengthening all our body systems we allow the body to 'fight back' against whatever has triggered the cognitive decline and avert the slide into dementia.

So one way of thinking about preventing MCI from developing into dementia might be to optimize – that is, to make the best of our health and well-being.

Generally, the holistic approach considers the following:

- diet (including nutritional supplements)
- exercise
- sleep
- brain exercise and stimulation
- addressing chronic health problems
- addressing inappropriate stress.

If you have read the previous chapters of this book you will quickly spot that all the areas addressed in the holistic approach have already been discussed. This is not really a radical approach; it is simply putting all the ideas about making the best of our health and well-being together.

When this kind of approach to health is mentioned I have sometimes heard people literally groan. Their feelings are that they are now well advanced in years, they have struggled to live a healthy life in the past, and that surely now they might be allowed a little latitude and be given leave to 'enjoy life'.

Whilst we all feel annoyed at times at the continuous 'healthy living' advice that is constantly preached by our doctors, by government agencies, by awareness groups and by the media, this should not mean that we give up and leave everything to fate. It may be sometimes irksome to watch our diet, to exercise more and to avoid things that are bad for our health, but in the whole time that I have supported people with dementia and their families, I have yet to meet anyone who describes having dementia as enjoyable or fun. So, if you want to 'enjoy life' in your senior years, it makes sense to do the things that will give you a longer life to enjoy. This is the very time of your life when you should be taking the most care of your health.

Some of those who advocate a holistic approach go further and try to suggest that Alzheimer's disease in particular can be divided into various 'types' and that the treatment should vary according to the type you have. The suggestion is that this also applies to MCI. The problem with this idea is that the suggested approach to discovering which type of cognitive problem you have involves a high number of tests, many of which are not readily available via a doctor in the UK.

What makes this approach significant is that it is highly personalized, targeted and multi-functional: the idea is not just to improve the status of the patient in each area, but also to 'optimize' it so that in every area of life the patient is achieving the very best status possible.

Most studies of this 'protocol' have been done in the USA. In the UK the restrictions of the National Health Service (NHS) mean that few people can obtain this kind of personalized targeted healthcare without paying for it, if they can find a practitioner who can deliver this approach at all.

This can seem very discouraging. What can make matters even more difficult is that if you approach your doctor and ask them to help you or to give you some information about how to optimize your health, you are likely to be disappointed.

First, doctors in the UK are very busy indeed, and are unlikely to have more than 10 minutes or so to discuss your problem with you. Second, very few doctors have much training in the intricacies of MCI and dementia. Third, given the knowledge that they do have, the things you are likely to be told will be very discouraging indeed. At one doctors' surgery where I was asked to visit and give the 'dementia specialist nurse' advice, I discovered that her protocols consisted of checking whether people with a dementia diagnosis had arranged a power of attorney (POA) and signed a 'Do Not Resuscitate' statement! Small wonder if patients decided that seeking advice from the surgery was a waste of time.

All this does not mean that if you happen to live in the UK and you have MCI you have to just give up and 'hope for the best'. Some things *are* within your control and you don't need the help of a doctor or expensive tests to manage certain health priorities.

Diet

As previously suggested, you can eat a good, varied diet. There are so many different lines of advice about diet currently that it is difficult to 'sort the wheat from the chaff'. You can at least try to follow some generally agreed guidelines if you have MCI. For example, most diet experts would suggest that it is particularly important to avoid too much 'processed' food. Cooking from scratch and making your own dishes from recipes doesn't have to use a lot of time. Often the best and most tasty and healthy meals are the simplest. For example, think about the following:

- baked potato with cheese, tuna or baked beans and salad
- shepherd's pie or cottage pie
- high-quality sausages, mashed potato and vegetables
- 'tray bakes' of chicken or fish and vegetables (cooked all together in the oven).

Avoid sugar if you can. It is easy to reduce a sweet tooth by cutting down slowly on your sugar intake. Sugar is addictive, so if you gradually cut it from your diet you will lose the taste for it and eventually even one chocolate or small piece of cake is 'too much'. Start by reducing any sugar that you take in tea and coffee by half a teaspoon at a time. After one week reduce it by another half teaspoon and so on, until you no longer need sugar in drinks. Then cut down on the number of biscuits or size of cake portion you eat. You will find that you still get the satisfaction of assuaging your sweet tooth with smaller portions. Try substituting yoghurt or fresh fruit for sweet cakes and biscuits.

There is some current research indicating that a period of 'fasting' of at least 12 hours between your last meal at night and your first meal in the morning can be beneficial for the brain. You could try this if it suits your lifestyle.[10]

Dietary supplements (vitamins and minerals)

There is a great deal of suggestion in the media that certain supplements may be 'good for the brain' and there is some truth in some of these claims. For example, a lack of some of the B vitamins can have an effect on memory and mental health. So, if you happen to be short of vitamin B and suffer from memory problems, taking a supplement to restore your levels of this vitamin will help your memory to function better. *But* if your vitamin B levels are within the normal range, then taking extra vitamin B will not help your memory.

Some people, particularly the elderly or those who do not go outside much or who keep themselves covered up, are frequently found to have low vitamin D levels. The best way to increase your level of vitamin D is to expose your skin to sunlight. But if you live in the extreme northern or southern hemisphere, where sunlight is in short supply, or in an areas where winters are dark and comparatively sunless, you can get your vitamin D from certain foods or from taking a supplement. It is not clear whether a lack of vitamin D has a direct effect on cognition, but some research seems to suggest that this is so.[11]

The same is true of the claims for many other supplements and for many other different foods. Some foods and some supplements do help the brain to function at its best, but whatever the media say, there are no actual 'superfoods'. The different dietary elements that are needed by the human body are found in many different foods, and the best way to ensure that we get all we need is to eat a wide range of foods.

However, if you feel that you need a vitamin supplement, it is unlikely to do you any harm to take one, provided you follow the guidelines given on the container and do not have more than the recommended dose. The same applies to any so-called 'superfoods'. It may do you good, and provided you use common sense about portions, it is unlikely to do you any harm.

Exercise

I have already pointed out that you do not need to go to the gym to exercise. Begin by just being a bit more active. Take a 10-minute walk every day. Increase this until you get to 20 minutes of brisk walking (about a mile). Do more of the exercise you enjoy, whether it is gardening, swimming, dancing or playing golf. If you would like to take up some form of exercise regime that will help to keep you supple and fit, then yoga, pilates and tai chi are all suitable.

It is possible to become more fit without a specific exercise routine just by making yourself more active every day. Make it a rule not to sit down for more than an hour at a time, and intersperse your sitting time with active time, even if this is only spent doing household chores or shopping. Keeping physically active can help too if you suffer from any form of rheumatism or arthritis. It is also important to do as much exercise as you can outdoors, and this brings us to the next recommendation.

One very important point that is often neglected by medical advisers is that you should get outside in the daylight as often as possible. Sometimes in the winter in some northern climates this can be a trial, but daylight is very important, and exercise in fresh air and daylight is the best there is.[12] Daylight can also have a very positive effect on sleep patterns and on depression.[13]

Sleep

Current research indicates that a good period (6–8 hours) of undisturbed sleep is very important in cutting the risk of developing dementia.[14] If you suffer from insomnia or disturbed nights, it is important to work out the reason and try to ensure a good night's sleep.

If you are disturbed by a sleeping partner – possibly because they need to get up to use the bathroom or because they snore or are otherwise restless – you may actually like to reconsider your sleeping arrangements. Many people have found that using a larger bed or twin beds rather than a double has helped their sleep pattern. Others find that they need to have separate bedrooms.

If you are disturbed because you need to use the bathroom yourself, then there are things you can try. Some people get up to use the toilet just because they are awake, but if you lie quietly and keep still you may find that you drift back to sleep. Try cutting down on the amount you drink in the hour or two before bed, but be careful not to get dehydrated. Sometimes your doctor can prescribe medication to help if you are frequently disturbed by the need for the toilet.

Sometimes people can be woken by pain; arthritis can be especially painful at night. Try to keep cool in bed as heat can exacerbate pain and so can constant restless movement. If your doctor prescribes medication for night-time pain, do not try to be 'brave' and avoid taking it – your sleep is very important.

If your sleep is disturbed by worries, there are a number of tactics you can try. Have a look at a helpful website such as that of the National Sleep Foundation,[15] and try out some of their suggestions.

It is generally recommended that you:

- sleep in a completely darkened room
- keep external noise to the minimum

- exclude TVs, electronic gadgets and mobile phones from your bedroom
- avoid using the above in the hour or two before bedtime
- go to bed at the same time each night.

One of my personal recommendations is to avoid checking emails or phone messages for at least a couple of hours before bed. If you receive a message that upsets you or needs you to take action, the subsequent worry can keep you awake. In the morning you will feel fresh and more able to deal with things.

Brain exercise and stimulation

It is not difficult to find numerous suggestions in the media that brain exercise is important. There are many books, websites, magazine articles and radio advertisements all suggesting that you should 'use it or lose it'. But what is the truth about so-called 'brain exercises'?

Some research has been carried out into the suggestion that we can improve our cognition by doing quizzes, crosswords, brain games and memory exercises. In general, crosswords, you will most probably get better at doing crosswords. But games, quizzes and memory exercises do not necessarily improve your general cognition. If you like doing these things, then do them because you like to do them. It is unlikely that doing them will prevent you getting dementia. Keeping your mind open to new ideas and being ready to try new activities and meet new people are things that are more likely to have a positive affect on your cognition. There is more information about this in Chapter 3.

If you have been told that you have MCI, you can take a conventional medical approach and just 'wait and see' or perhaps 'wait and hope'. If you wish to be more proactive, you can address any immediate and obvious health issues and high-risk factors, and this is a sensible pathway. However, you have nothing to lose and perhaps everything to gain by concentrating on a holistic approach and doing all you can to ensure that your body and brain are functioning at optimum level. Even if you cannot follow the highly personalized protocols suggested by some practitioners, there are many things you can do to take control of your own health and to secure the best cognitive future possible.

Key points

- At present we do not know why some people with MCI progress to dementia, but reducing dementia risk factors is worthwhile.
- Dementia is thought to start long before symptoms manifest themselves.
- If you have MCI, most conventional practitioners take a 'wait and see' approach.
- You can take self-help measures at any time.
- A holistic approach to your health is likely to have the most beneficial effect.

Endnotes

1   Tomaszewski Farias, S., Mungas, D., Reed, B.R., Harvey, D. and DeCarli, C. (2009) 'Progression of mild cognitive impairment to dementia in clinic- vs community-based cohorts.' *JAMA Neurology* 66, 9, 1151–1157. Available at https://jamanetwork.com/journals/jamaneurology/fullarticle/797955

2   Livingston, G., Sommerlad, A., Orgeta, V., Costafreda, S.G., *et al.* (2017) 'Dementia prevention, intervention and care.' *The Lancet* 390, 10113.

3   Velayudhan, L., Poppe, M., Archer, N., Proitsi, P., Brown, R.G. and Lovestone, S. (2010) 'Risk of developing dementia in people with diabetes and mild cognitive impairment.' *British Journal of Psychiatry* 196, 1, 36–40.

4   Asif, M. (2014) 'The prevention and control of type-2 diabetes by changing lifestyle and dietary pattern.' *Journal of Education and Health Promotion* 3, 1. doi:10.4103/2277-9531.127541

5   Lin, F.R., Ferrucci, L., An, Y., Goh, J.O., *et al.* (2014) 'Association of hearing impairment with brain volume changes in older adults.' *Neuroimage* 90, 84–92. doi:10.106/j.neuroimage.2013.12.059

6   Justin, B.N., Turek, M. and Hakim, A.M. (2013) 'Heart disease as a risk factor for dementia.' *Clinical Epidemiology* 5, 135–145. doi:10.2147/CLEP.S30621

7   Bredesen, D.E., Sharlin, K., Jenkins, D., Okuno, M., *et al.* (2018) 'Reversal of cognitive decline: 100 patients.' *Journal of Alzheimer's Disease and Parkinsonism* 8, 450. doi:10.4172/2161-0460.1000450

8   Myhill, S. (2015) *Sustainable Medicine*. London: Hammersmith Health Books.

9   Ibid, p.205.

10 Youm, Y.-H., Nguyen, K.Y., Grant, R.W., Goldberg, E.L., *et al.* (2015) 'The ketone metabolite β-hydroxybutyrate blocks NLRP3 inflammasome-mediated inflammatory disease.' *Nature Medicine* 21, 263–269. doi:10.1038/nm.3804

11 Lu'o'ng, K.V.Q. and Nguyen, L.T.H. (2011) 'The beneficial role of vitamin D in Alzheimer's disease.' *American Journal of Alzheimer's Disease and Other Dementias* 26, 7, 511–520. doi:10.1177/1533317511429321

12 Aries, M.B.C., Aarts, M.P.J. and van Hoof, J. (2013) 'Daylight and health: A review of the evidence and consequences for the built environment.' *Lighting Research & Technology* 47, 1. Available at https://doi.org/10.1177/1477153513509258

13 Buysse, D.J. (2014) 'Sleep health: Can we define it? Does it matter?' *Sleep* 37, 1, 9–17. doi:10.5665/sleep.3298

14 Shokri-Kojori, E., Wang, G.-J., Wiers, C.E., Demiral, S.B., *et al.* (2018) 'β-Amyloid accumulation in the human brain after one night of sleep deprivation.' *PNAS: Proceedings of the National Academy of Sciences* 115, 17, 4483–4488. Available at www.pnas.org/content/early/2018/03/29/1721694115.full

15 www.sleepfoundation.org

Chapter 9

If the Worst Should Happen...Planning in the Event of a Dementia Diagnosis

This book is about mild cognitive impairment (MCI) and about how to help yourself if you have a mild cognitive problem that is not dementia. A good part of the book has discussed how to try to prevent MCI from developing into dementia. However, evidence indicates that a percentage of people with MCI do go on to develop dementia. Robust figures are hard to find; suggested 'conversion rates' vary from 5–10 per cent[1] to about 48 per cent,[2] and some researchers have posited that MCI is simply early dementia in disguise.[3] So what do you do if the worst should happen?

Is it the worst that can happen?

You might start by asking yourself if this is 'the worst that can happen'. Dementia is an unpleasant and progressive disease and many of us dread it. But the surprising thing is that many people who actually have a diagnosis of dementia are not intrinsically unhappy. People with dementia may be frustrated that they can no longer do the things that they used to do and sometimes dementia is accompanied by depression (although it is not necessarily the cause of the depression), but after the first frustrating and difficult months, many people with dementia seem to be almost serene. It is possibly the fact that they no longer have to cope with all the minor pinpricks of life – the washing machine breaking down, the car needing servicing, the shopping needing doing – because someone else takes these things over and they no longer cause worry to the person with dementia. We just do not know.

Of course, not everyone with dementia is happy and serene, but those who are not living alone and whose partners in life are supportive and kind often do develop a kind of calm peacefulness. Most often, dementia is pain-free as well, and although carers will have to endure the degeneration of physical abilities as the brain deteriorates, they will not have to witness a loved one in pain whilst feeling unable to help.

It is often believed that dementia shortens life and doctors are prone to quoting an 'average' lifespan of seven years from diagnosis. However, it must be remembered that for many people, the diagnosis only happens when they are quite elderly and perhaps already infirm in some other way. The odds are surely that the 'seven-year average' is no more than the lifespan that someone of this age and infirmity would expect in any case.

I am not trying to suggest that you should be happy and glad about such a diagnosis, but some aspects are less daunting then we might fear. For one thing, the progress of dementia is usually (but not always) fairly gradual and you may have some months, if not years, of life to enjoy with only minor adjustments before things become difficult.

A diagnosis also gives the chance to plan for the future and if, perhaps, you have been putting off some plan for a 'lifetime experience', this can be the very time to take advantage of the opportunity to take the plunge and enjoy the experience without worrying whether you are doing the right thing.

Review your plans and actions

Parts of this book have been about making plans for the future and this is a good time and opportunity to review those plans. In many ways, if you or your loved one have experienced MCI, you will have had an opportunity to take a step back and look at where you are going in life, a chance to plan ahead or at least to take a long cool look at what might lie ahead, and a chance to review your current and future needs and your need for support in the future.

Hopefully, if you have taken notice of previous advice in this book, your plans will have incorporated thinking about:

- Practical matters like power of attorney (POA), wills and other financial advice.
- Health matters like attention to diet and exercise, paying attention to eyesight and hearing problems,

avoiding unnecessary surgery, coping with and containing infections, and choosing healthcare advisers wisely.

- Moving home if necessary, before a crisis happens, talking about the future with your family, drawing up end-of-life care plans and using technology to help you manage everyday life.
- Using memory aids to manage activities of daily living.
- Potential support from family and friends.

Think of yourself as one of the lucky people: due to your knowledge and understanding of MCI, you and your loved one have had the opportunity to think ahead and consider a future that most people prefer to avoid thinking about. If you have followed the advice in this book, you will already have considered the possibility of moving home; drawn up plans for future support; and researched the healthy advice from care agencies and local services. You will also have already bought or obtained memory aids that can help maintain independence (and discarded those you have found of no practical use). People who have a diagnosis of dementia thrust upon them suddenly have all this to deal with. You have already dealt with it. Haven't you?

Practical steps

It is essential to arrange lasting power of attorney (LPA) now if you have not yet done so. Remember that when you give POA to someone, you are giving them the power to take decisions about your finances, your health and your welfare if you become unable to make these decisions yourself. Many situations can raise a need for this, not only dementia. If, for example, you have an accident or are taken ill and are unable to express your wishes, then someone who has POA will be empowered to act on your behalf. If you have not done it before (see Chapter 2), this is a good moment to have frank discussions with the family. You may believe that you and they feel the same about something such as resuscitation, assisted suicide or residential care homes, but once you begin to talk about these subjects, you may be surprised. Make sure that your own personal feelings are known, and if you are the carer of someone with dementia, help to ensure that their wishes are known and carried out.

The same applies to wishes about end of life. It really is no good pushing these discussions aside as too painful unless you have no strong feelings about the matter. If you do not wish to be resuscitated in an extreme situation, you need to write this down and make sure that your family know about it. If you are caring for a spouse who has been diagnosed with dementia, and if you have previously discussed these difficult matters with them, be sure to make their wishes known to the family and to medical advisers. It is really important if you have a spouse or partner or perhaps a parent who has now been diagnosed with dementia, to consider what they would actually want *and not what you, in their shoes, think you would want*. If they are still able to write their wishes down, assist them to do so.

Just because someone has dementia does not mean that they are incapable of making a will. However, as usual, we have to consider the matter of 'capacity'. In the early stages of dementia most people understand what making a will means and would be able to indicate what they would like to happen to their estate after they die. If someone with dementia wants to make a will, it is possible that they can still do so given the right support and explanations. Most of us do not draw up our wills ourselves (although such wills are normally perfectly valid) – we use an 'expert' to do this for us. Someone with dementia can also use an 'expert' to draw up the will, and provided that they have capacity (that is, understanding) of what their decisions signify, they can make a valid decision about this.

Health matters

Dementia is a physical illness that has an effect on the brain. It is more important than ever that someone with dementia takes care of their general health. In most cases, they will need someone else – their primary carer – to help them with this. In previous chapters we have looked in some depth at the need to optimize eyesight, hearing and general health, and we have also looked at diet and the effect this might have on the brain.

Frequently (but not inevitably) people with dementia lose weight, and usually carers and health professionals are at a loss to explain this. Henry Lorin, in his book *Alzheimer's Solved*,[4] gives a suggested and plausible explanation for this weight loss – that low cholesterol is at the root of the problem. Most health professionals would not agree with him, as current thinking is still preoccupied with the suggestion that cholesterol is to blame for heart disease, but Lorin suggests that low cholesterol is responsible for the weight loss of people with dementia. Whatever the explanation, the fact is that those people with dementia who suffer from weight loss generally continue to have a normal appetite, and carers can become very concerned about how to help. The most important thing is to ensure that the person with dementia eats a diet that is nutritionally sound. There is further information about this in Chapter 3, and if you are now confronting a diagnosis of dementia, I recommend that you read that chapter again.

Of course, as dementia progresses, the person with dementia becomes less able to make their own health decisions – decisions such as whether to have minor or major surgery, which medicines to take and how to take them, and which medical advisers to choose and when to consult them. The primary carer must help them to make these decisions and, as the disease progresses, must make these decisions on their behalf. It is important for the carer to familiarize themselves with the risks and benefits of such decisions, and these may change once a diagnosis has been made. For example, it may be unwise to have a general anaesthetic in some cases of dementia. If a necessary general anaesthetic is administered, it is worth remembering that dementia may make confusion and loss of cognition worse in the days after a surgical operation. People with dementia may also become less able to express that they feel unwell or that they are in pain, so the primary carer must again be more vigilant in noticing changes in behaviour that might indicate this. In particular, a urinary or chest infection – indeed, any infection, even the common

cold – may cause the person with dementia to exhibit
more confusion or more difficult behaviour than usual.
Many of my clients have realized belatedly that unusual
stubbornness, agitation or aggression can be the herald
of illness.

Moving home

Many of my clients are diagnosed shortly after moving
home. This does not mean that moving home caused the
dementia, but rather that having to find new networks,
learning new routes and beginning new routines
exacerbates and highlights the difficulties that were already
being experienced. So, is it a good idea to move home
having been diagnosed with dementia?

As with many decisions, this depends on a number
of factors. In my experience people who already have a
diagnosis of dementia will get worse (sometimes only
temporarily) after the move because of the difficulty
of learning new routines, new routes and making new
networks of friends and neighbours. However, other factors
may outweigh this. For example, you may wish to be nearer
to family and support networks or you may need to find a
house or flat that is smaller, easier to manage and better
equipped.

Bear in mind that if you move to be nearer family, you
will still need to make your own new friends, get to know
your neighbours and learn your way around the area. It is a
very bad idea to rely solely on nearby families for support
– they may not have the time or the capacity to give you

all the support you need. In any case, you would not wish to burden them with responsibility for all the support you may need.

Another factor to consider is the change of medical professionals. If you found the diagnostic process smooth and you are receiving lots of support in the place you live, it may be a shock to discover that a new doctor is less knowledgeable or sympathetic or that there are no activities or groups in the new area that are suitable for people who have a dementia diagnosis.

If you do move house following a diagnosis, expect problems with confusion and forgetfulness that may last longer than you anticipate. Take the time to ensure that the person with dementia is given the chance to learn new routes around the area. For example, do not just drive them everywhere – find local shops and amenities and help them to learn how to get to these. You will find that it is likely that they will need a lot longer to learn their way about and you may have to take them on a number of 'guided' walks around the neighbourhood before they are confident. It is possible that the person with dementia may forget where they live, and if you have not moved far, they may journey back to their old address in error sometimes.

Accept support – build a team

When I am asked what is the single most important piece of advice I can give to people who are beginning to live with dementia (and this includes carers and the family of the person diagnosed), I will always say it is to *accept support*.

Many people are very reluctant to accept support or to ask for help and the reasons for this are discussed in earlier chapters. But I believe very firmly that you cannot cope alone with dementia.

If you are living with someone who has just been diagnosed, you may think that this statement is quite wrong. This is because you are living in the present and are unable to project your thoughts into the future and to understand thoroughly what living with dementia, as it progresses, really means. I do understand this, and I do try frequently to explain to my new clients about progression and to give them, as clearly as I can, a picture of what the effects of the dementia will be.

Dementia is relentless, and if you live with someone who has dementia it is with you all day and every day. As the disease progresses the person with dementia becomes less and less able to do even simple tasks alone without supervision. Carers need respite time – time to enjoy their own interests and time to rest (see pp.190-3). There are many kinds of respite; having a friend, neighbour or family member take the person you care for down to the pub for a drink or out shopping for clothes is one kind. Making use of a day centre to give yourself time to visit the bank, have a haircut or do some shopping yourself is another. Paying a care agency to help your cared-for with washing and dressing is another type of respite. In the immediate time after diagnosis you may balk at the idea that you will ever need some of these kinds of support, but the odds are that you will.

All this sounds very depressing, but the people who manage best after diagnosis and who manage to live well with dementia and to keep a good quality of life are those who make use of all the support they can. The early days are the time to build your 'team' of supporters so that when things progress you can put help into place with the minimum of fuss and the least difficulty. Even if you are convinced that you will never need any of this kind of support, I urge you to find out what is available, make a note of the contacts you might need and be better prepared for the time ahead.

What treatment is there?

The hardest part of the diagnosis of dementia is the realization that medical help is strictly limited for this condition. We are so used to the concept that many illnesses can be cured and that those for which there is at present no cure (such as diabetes) can at least be 'managed' by medical means. It is very difficult to come to terms with the fact that medical science still has no real means of either curing or 'managing' dementia. It is true that the media are every day proclaiming that a 'cure has been found' or a breakthrough has been made, but read below the beguiling headlines and you will see that this is just not true.

More than a decade ago some drugs became available that were found, in some cases, to slow the progress of dementia for a limited time. This is what the drugs are and what they do. Three of the so-called 'memory drugs' work in a similar way. They are cholinesterase inhibitors, and some people taking these drugs are reported to experience improvements in motivation, anxiety levels and confidence and an increased ability to deal with the tasks of everyday living as well as improved memory. Not everyone notices an improvement and some people find the side effects of the drugs unacceptable. Symptoms are likely to improve only temporarily, although more recent research has indicated that the drugs continue to be beneficial, even in late dementia.[5] The important thing to remember, however, is that the drugs do not stop the progression of dementia.

The fourth drug commonly given in dementia is an NDMA (N-methyl-D-aspartate) receptor, and this is sometimes given along with one of the cholinesterase inhibitors. This drug can help with symptoms of aggression and agitation and can temporarily slow progression of the symptoms; side effects are reported less commonly.

There is some evidence that certain 'self-help' activities can make a difference. They may slow the progression of symptoms and are usually acknowledged to make the person with dementia feel better about themselves and to suffer less depression and loss of confidence. These non-medical interventions are also good for general health:

- *Exercise:* any exercise is better than none. You do not have to join a gym – even walking is good for you. Exercise helps our cardiovascular health (it's good for your heart, in other words), and there is some limited evidence that it also improves cognition. In this respect physical exercise is thought to be of more use than so-called 'brain exercise' (doing crosswords and puzzles). Physical exercise will also help to retain fitness and balance and may help to prevent falls, which are one of the most frequent causes of hospital admission in the elderly.

- *Being socially active:* there is more evidence that keeping active socially is helpful. Many people with dementia begin to withdraw from their normal social circle because they find it difficult to keep up with conversation or because they feel less comfortable in large groups. In fact, many of my clients have said that they noticed the social withdrawal beginning even before diagnosis. But social activity – as long as it does not cause undue stress – is good for people with dementia. So, if you have someone in the family who has now been diagnosed with dementia, help them to keep up their activities and find ways to ensure that this is not stressful for them.

- *Cognitive Stimulation Therapy* (CST): this is a specific therapy that is recommended by NICE (National Institute for Health and Care Excellence) for those in early stage dementia. If it is available and is offered to you, try it out.

- *Music and singing:* this has been shown time and again to have a mood-lifting effect and to help the memory of those with dementia. There are now a number of 'Singing for the Brain' and 'Singing for the Mind' groups, but if someone who has been diagnosed with dementia is already a member of a choir or singing group, then help them to keep up this activity as long as possible.

- *Memory aids*: all the suggestions for using memory aids and equipment to make life easier which are referred to in Chapter 6 will also be of use. Some memory aids only work in early dementia, but the earlier someone gets used to them, the longer they seem to be of use.

You will find a lot more information about 'self-help' measures in Chapter 5 of this book. In general, activities which help prevent dementia and which are recommended for MCI are also beneficial in the early stages of the disease.

Find your way around health and social care

After a diagnosis you suddenly find yourself finding out about health and social care. Perhaps you have got used to the health system because of another long-standing health problem. If this is the case you may have a head start. If you have generally remained healthy until now, you may be surprised to find that you will now be 'absorbed' into the system. Every area is different – there is no standard 'dementia pathway', although many health authorities use that term. It is very likely that following diagnosis you will be offered some follow-up support. This may take any of the following forms:

- A visit (or visits) from a dementia specialist, usually a nurse, to supervise the issue of any memory medication, deal with any side effects and arrange changes in dosage, where necessary.

- A follow-up (or follow-ups) by your doctor or a general practice-trained nurse specializing in dementia follow-up. This will usually take place at the doctors' surgery and may seem to concentrate on physical measures such as blood pressure and weight or blood tests rather than any support.

- Offer of a place on a post-diagnostic 'course', sometimes called 'memory matters' or a 'memory clinic', or some other name. This is a useful option, and if it is offered, I advise you to take it up. This kind of course will take you through the immediate problems likely to be encountered, and will enable you to think about the future and make plans for when the disease progresses. A sensible idea is to take notes during this course as you may find there is a lot of information given, although some of it you will not need immediately.

- A referral to social care (see below).

- A referral (or contact information) to local and national support organizations such as Age UK, Alzheimer's Society, Action for Carers, Citizens Advice, and any local support such as dementia cafes, cognitive stimulation groups or carers support groups. At this stage you may feel that you do not need any of these, but it is wise to make a note of the details because you will be glad to know about them in due course.

Social care

Most of us are aware that there is a social care system in our country. In the UK everyone is entitled to free advice from social care, and some people will be entitled to free services provided by the social care team. You may think that you are entitled to more than the social care team offer or you may think that you do not need their services. It is wise to find out what is available in your area and to be aware in what circumstances you may call on their help. In some areas doctors are very knowledgeable and active in involving social care when it is needed. In other cases it seems to be up to the individual to seek help in this area. You can self-refer to social services and you do not have to wait until someone thinks you need help to investigate what is available.

Be aware that although free help from social care is means tested and only available to those on a low income, everyone, whether they qualify for free help or not, is entitled to free advice and information. Chapter 10 gives further information about how to get help and which organizations are available in individual cases.

Carer - care for yourself

This particular section of the chapter is directed at the person most directly responsible for providing help and support for a person diagnosed with dementia. These people are usually referred to as 'the carer'. You may not like this term or wish to use it, but nevertheless, it is a commonly accepted and understood term and is used in most information literature and media concerned with dementia.

If you are this person – the carer of someone with dementia – it is important to keep in mind that you should be aware of your own well-being. If a diagnosis has just been made, you may feel that thinking about yourself is not very important just now, and that it is more important to consider the well-being and health of the one you care for.

You are going to find that time to yourself will soon be in short supply. This is not meant to frighten you but only to help you understand. Initially someone with early stage dementia just needs a little help – perhaps a few memory aids, a written list, a well-organized calendar and a 'nudge' from you (the primary carer) every now and again.

But dementia is progressive, and the thing most people fail to understand in the early days is the *way* in which dementia affects the working of the brain. It is not just a case of giving people a little help to remember or writing out a list of more easily understood instructions. Dementia attacks the heart of a person's ability and understanding. The person with dementia becomes unable to understand what things are used for, how to begin and proceed with a task, where to go to find everyday items and who other people are in relation to themselves. Eventually it isn't just a case of reminding someone to clean their teeth: it is showing them where the bathroom is, turning on the taps for them, placing the toothpaste on the brush and probably actually cleaning their teeth for them because they no longer understand what they have to do.

Multiply that description of a small hygiene task by all the things we have to do just to function in this life, and you may begin to understand what is ahead of you.

Probably more difficult to understand and to deal with is the fact that as time proceeds, the person with dementia will become unable to entertain themselves. This means that they will not be able to read a book to pass the time (the ability to read often remains, but in order to enjoy reading a book you have to be able to remember what you read on the page before), go for a walk alone (in case they lose their way), do the shopping (they will not remember what they are shopping for or how to handle money), carry out a hobby, do mundane chores or even in some cases watch TV (some people with dementia enjoy certain TV programmes but they can no longer follow a plot).

What I am trying to explain is that as time progresses, people with dementia need someone with them *all the time*.

Because an increasingly heavy burden falls on the primary carer, it is very important that this carer cares for themselves. First, you should take care of your own health. Remember that if something happens to you – sickness, a hospital stay, a fall or an accident – the person you are caring for will have to be looked after. This may mean a confusing stay at a relative's or in a residential care home because they will not be able to stay at home alone. Remember, too, that they will not be able to look after you if you fall ill. Of course no one can mitigate against every unforeseen circumstance, but you can at least take care to eat properly, to get enough sleep and to have any regular medical check-ups that are advised.

You should also plan for some respite time – some time you can call your own when you can pursue your own hobbies or interests, take care of routine maintenance matters and enjoy not being 'on call'. There is more about this earlier in the chapter, discussed under 'Accept support'.

There are carers support organizations that can help: support groups that enable you to meet others in the same situation; clubs and cafes where you can go with your cared-for; and even organizations that arrange holidays that you and your cared-for can enjoy together, where care and support is provided as well as entertainment.

You can find out more about all sources of support and help in Chapter 10.

Key points

- A dementia diagnosis need not be devastating.
- If you have read this book and taken the actions suggested, you are already prepared.
- Review your plans and put into action anything that needs doing now.
- Find out about support and be prepared to accept it.
- Investigate medication and therapy.
- Familiarize yourself about health and social care professionals.
- If you are a carer, take care of yourself.

Endnotes

1   Mitchell, A.J. and Shiri-Feshki, M. (2009) 'Rate of progression of mild cognitive impairment to dementia – meta-analysis of 41 robust inception cohort studies.' *Acta Psychiatrica Scandinavica* 119, 4, 252–265. doi:10.1111/j.1600-0447.2008.01326.x

2   Fischer, P., Jungwirth, S., Zehetmayer, S., Weissgram, S., *et al.* (2007) 'Conversion from subtypes of mild cognitive impairment to Alzheimer dementia.' *Neurology* 68, 4, 288–291.

3   Bruscoli, M. and Lovestone, S. (2004) 'Is MCI really just early dementia? Asystematic review of conversion studies.' *International Psychogeriatrics* 16, 2, 129–140. doi:10.1017/S1041610204000092

4   Lorin, H. (2006) *Alzheimer's Solved (Condensed Edition)*. CreateSpace Independent Publishing Platform.

5   Livingston, G., Sommerlad, A., Orgeta, V., Costafreda, S.G., *et al.* (2017) 'Dementia prevention, intervention and care.' *The Lancet* 390, 10113.

Chapter 10

Sources of Help, Advice and Support

Many people are reluctant to ask for or accept help, and this seems to apply especially when it comes to cognitive problems (that is, difficulties with memory). This may be because it feels demeaning to be asking for help and support to manage confusion or slowness. The same people who would prefer to manage alone when it comes to a cognitive problem would probably not have the same difficulty if they needed help because of a physical difficulty. Few of us would refuse to use a crutch if we have broken a leg, for example, or to make use of a lift if we have trouble climbing stairs due to a disabling condition such as arthritis.

Many people are determined to be independent and to 'manage'. I used to see this when I helped to run a diagnostic clinic alongside a consultant psychiatrist who specialized in the health of older people. Our clinic was specifically concerned with dementia. Those who had been referred to the clinic with memory problems who were then given a diagnosis of dementia were always referred immediately to the support service I was providing.

A few welcomed the opportunity to ask questions and get information about the condition, but many put me off – 'Thank you, but we can manage at the moment. We will ask for help when we need it.' Of course everyone has the right to refuse help, but it seemed to me that many turned down the offer of support because they were unable to recognize that they would need it sooner or later. Most of those who refused support returned later to the service, but it was frustrating to know that support and information can be of most use early in dementia and also frustrating only to be asked to provide it when things had reached crisis stage.

But what of those who did not receive a diagnosis? A few people were identified as having a specific medical condition that was not dementia and that could be treated or even cured once they were referred to the right speciality.

Others were identified as having mild cognitive impairment (MCI). They would be reassured that there was no diagnosis of dementia – that they might get better spontaneously or after some other medical condition that was affecting their cognition was treated. They might remain the same: their MCI would remain but would not progress to dementia. However, there was always a warning that the condition might progress and in one or two years or sooner they might indeed receive the dreaded diagnosis.

Usually these people would ask what they could do to help themselves. Usually they were given general advice about keeping to a healthy lifestyle and 'to go on as they were'. If symptoms seemed to get worse and they were worried, they could come back at a later date.

As my remit was dementia and not MCI, I was not allowed to give advice to these people because they did not have a dementia diagnosis. If I could have given advice, I would have pointed them to sources of support and information, such as those given below.

Accepting support does not necessarily mean speaking to an adviser. Not everyone wants this kind of one-to-one contact. Support, advice and information can all be obtained from many sources. This book is one kind of support (and I hope you are finding it useful). You may prefer to look at online sources of information, and most organizations have a website you can access. Some people still prefer to go to a central place – such as the local public library – to access information. Some would indeed prefer to speak to an adviser face-to-face or on the telephone. There are also more informal local sources such as dementia cafes, community support groups and social groups not specifically aimed at MCI but where you may find appropriate help.

Sources of support for those with MCI are not obvious. You might like to consider your individual problems, such as short-term memory loss, difficulty in managing certain life areas, or problems with route finding, and look for specific support for that particular area.

Aids and equipment to help with everyday living

Independent Living: This organization provides impartial information about living independently with a disability. They are not part of a charity or government organization. They provide information on products and services and users can sign up to a weekly email news round-up. They do not deal exclusively with memory problems or dementia-related issues, but there is plenty of information about these. They have a dedicated website area for cognitive issues:

www.independentliving.co.uk/il-editorials/dementia-cognitive-impairment

Advice and support for cognitive problems

Alzheimer's Society: This is a registered charity operating within England, Wales and Northern Ireland. It provides information and raises money for research into all types of dementia. There is also a 'hands-on' support service that helps people who have a dementia diagnosis. Different levels of service are provided in different areas depending on funding. Normally services are not offered to people without an 'official' diagnosis of some form of dementia, but information on the website is accessible to anyone. There are links to other services:

www.alzheimers.org.uk

Alzheimer Scotland: The leading dementia organization in Scotland:

www.alzscot.org

Other advice and support, including financial advice

Citizens Advice: A network of independent charities offering confidential advice online, over the

telephone, and in person, free of charge. They claim to
be independent and totally impartial. They give advice on
consumer rights and pension guidance[1] to people aged over 50.
You can check their website, visit one of their local centres in
person or obtain advice via telephone on a range of problems.
If they do not actually deal with the specific problem you
have, they will direct you to a service that can help:

www.citizensadvice.org.uk

Age UK: They have a range of support, advice and
information available about money and legal matters, health
in older life and care and support. You can find out more
from their website. They also offer local services such as
foot care, a handyman service, dementia support, shopping
and social activities. The range of services available varies
in different places so it is best to enquire locally or you
can search their website to find what is available to you in
your area:

www.ageuk.org.uk/services/in-your-area

Information about paying for care

Independent Age: This organization provides clear, free
and impartial advice on care and support, money and
benefits and health and mobility:

www.independentage.org

Care Information Scotland: Offers information if you look after someone, need care yourself or are planning for future care needs:

www.careinfoscotland.scot

Wills

There are several websites and books that will help with writing a will, such as:

www.gov.uk/make-will

Power of attorney (POA)

The procedures and rules about power of attorney (POA) are complicated, and although you can draw up a POA yourself (you can download a form or send for a form to complete), many people prefer to get a solicitor to do the work for them. You can get information and download the forms from the government website:

www.gov.uk/power-of-attorney

Driving

Statistics show that older people are not necessarily more prone to motor accidents and nor are they less able drivers. It is thought that driving experience and care compensate for the sharper reactions that younger drivers may have. However, many older drivers feel less confident when driving on routes that they do not know well, and it is likely that older drivers are not so familiar with changes recently introduced to the Highway Code. If you feel that you need a confidence boost or that you would just like reassurance that your driving skills are up to scratch, several organizations can help. Rather than approaching a traditional driving instructor for refresher lessons it might be worth taking an assessment specifically designed with older drivers in mind. Most of the organizations that offer such assessments stress that they offer a one-to-one confidential assessment and that they do not notify any third party of the result. So you can take the opportunity to check out your driving skills without feeling that you are being 'tested'. Some organizations such as the **Royal Society for the Prevention of Accidents** (RoSPA) or **IAM RoadSmart** (formerly the institute of Advanced Motorists) operate in all parts of the country, whilst many local councils run driver assessment schemes in their own areas. You will normally have to pay for such an assessment:

www.roadar.org.uk/drivers/driving-assessments.htm

www.iamroadsmart.com/courses/mature-driver-review

If you are involved in a motor accident, the police can sometimes insist that you take a driving assessment. Similarly, if you are caught exceeding the speed limit, you may be offered a chance to attend a speed awareness course instead of paying a fine. In either case it is worth accepting the opportunity to attend an assessment or course as you may learn how to improve your driving.

Other methods of transport

People over 60 in the UK are eligible for a bus pass that gives them free travel within certain hours. Some local authorities also allow travel in the morning rush hour and in some areas passes can also be used on trams, trains or taxis. Bus passes are issued by local councils so check your local council website or ask at the council office to find if you are eligible for this.

Many local councils run a low-cost door-to-door minibus service. You will usually have to register for this service and there will be a charge, but the benefit is that you get door-to-door service and the vehicles are suitable for frail or disabled people. Check with your local council or your local public library to find out details of what is available.

There are many local community transport services that use volunteer drivers. Again, you will need to check locally what is available. To use this service you usually need to book in advance and a small contribution towards fuel costs is expected, but as above, you get a door-to-door service.

For those who prefer to pay privately, it is worth checking for services such as **Driving Miss Daisy**. This is what they say on their website:

We provide transportation and companion driving services for the elderly, children, disabled and for anyone who is unable to drive from A to B. We offer you independence and peace of mind, enabling you to get out, have fun, and add some zing into your everyday living. Our special service also provides assistance in and out of the car, going to appointments, shopping and company on outings.

Special needs are catered for including assistance with a walker [Zimmer frame] or wheelchair.

https://drivingmissdaisy.co.uk

Brain plasticity

Despite the many claims made by 'brain game' manufacturers, there is at present no evidence to prove that playing brain games actually helps to improve cognition. The general consensus is that if you play a game often, you will get better, but only at playing that particular game. The same goes for doing crosswords and other word puzzles. If you enjoy doing these things, then by all means continue to do them, but it is unlikely that they will improve your brain power on their own.

However, it is thought that you can continue to improve your brain plasticity (see Chapter 5) in later life by enjoying new activities and experiences and by learning new skills. Here are some sources of information and ideas, but really, learning anything new is probably of benefit, so this list is not exclusive.

Learning a new language: many books and audio courses are available as well as conventional 'evening classes'. In many areas the **University of the Third Age** (U3A) run conversation classes in different languages. If you enjoy online games, try:

www.duolingo.com

Learning a new subject: some people find the cost of classes a problem; a good free source of learning is:

www.futurelearn.com

Learning a musical instrument or singing in a choir: Music is relaxing, therapeutic and entertaining, and singing is known to enhance memory. There are a number of 'Singing for the Brain' groups in the UK, and this service is organized by the Alzheimer's Society. But there are also many music groups, community choirs and 'Singing for Fun' groups. It may be worth looking at what is organized by your local council. If you are interested in music rather than singing, again, see what is available locally in the way of music appreciation groups. Music is one area where you can enjoy the benefits in your own home simply by listening to the radio, a CD or downloading music on your internet device:

www.alzheimers.org.uk/get-support/your-support-services/singing-for-the-brain

www.singforfun.co.uk

https://communitychoirsuk.com

If, despite all the suggestions above, you would really like to try some online brain games, the following are worth looking at:

www.memory-improvement-tips.com/brain-games.html

www.lumosity.com/en

Recovery from stroke

Stroke can have a devastating effect on an individual but it is worth remembering that many people make a good recovery and can learn to use their limbs again, improve their speech if it has been affected and make use of the 'plasticity' of the brain to relearn many of the abilities that were lost due to the stroke:

www.stroke.org.uk

The **Stroke Association** (website above) runs local support services in many areas and the website offers information and support.

A useful and very detailed book for anyone wanting to work hard at their own recovery is: **Janet Carr and Roberta Shepherd** (2003) *Stroke Rehabilitation – Guidelines for Exercise and Training to Optimize Motor Skill*, published by Elsevier.

Social care

If you feel that you need help from the social care team (what most people mean when they refer to 'social services'), contact your local council's social services department for a care needs assessment. Bear in mind that any help provided is subject to a means test and you may have to pay for some or all of the cost. You can find out the local contact for social care from your local council website or through the local library or Citizens Advice.

Financial matters, including paying for care

Paying for care is a major factor in the many decisions that have to be taken as we age. I know from discussions with clients that this is one of the most difficult areas to address. There are two sides to this. The first is the fact that many people do not feel that they should have to pay for care if their need is due to dementia. This is a very valid argument because dementia is a physical illness, and yet the government treats care needs in dementia as purely a 'social need'.

The second factor is the high cost of care, particularly residential care. Even though care providers can give a good account and adequate breakdown of costs and show how the costs are calculated, the monies involved still seem outrageous. Residential care costs can eat into savings very quickly.

Some people plan ahead for the possibility of care being needed in the future. There are a number of firms that specialize in helping people to plan for this contingency. You can get advice from many private sources about organizing your finances to take into account care costs. If you are concerned about care home fees and continuing healthcare, check out:

https://caretobedifferent.co.uk

The government **Money Advice Service** gives a range of information about money matters including care costs:

www.moneyadviceservice.org.uk

Citizens Advice (see pp.198–199) can give help with financial problems such as debts, pensions and access to benefits.

Age UK (see p.199) also offers free useful advice about care costs.

The government has a general website with information on benefits:

www.gov.uk/browse/benefits

Everyday living

Older people need to be more aware of the risk of falls and accidents, and people with MCI should take extra care. As pointed out in earlier chapters of this book, falls are a major cause of hospitalization and future frailty. Many falls happen in the home, so it is worth checking or having someone else check over your home with you to minimize risks for falls. Even something as simple as improving lighting can make a big difference. This website gives some useful tips:

www.healthinaging.org/tools-and-tips/home-safety-tips-older-adults

The **Royal Society for the Prevention of Accidents** (RoSPA) also has useful information:

www.rospa.com/Home-Safety

Some people are eligible for a free assessment of the home from an **occupational therapist** – your doctor can advise if you are eligible for this. If you cannot get a free assessment you can pay for a professional assessment and this may be worthwhile. The aim of occupational therapists is to help people to function as independently as possible:

https://rcotss-ip.org.uk/what-is-occupational-therapy

Some local councils run low-cost or free courses for senior adults that help improve their balance and freedom of movement. Similar courses are also offered by local leisure centres and gyms. There are many initiatives in different areas concerned with safety and with falls prevention. The best thing to do is enquire at your local public library, doctors' surgery or Citizens Advice to see what is available in your area.

In some areas, **Action for Carers** run courses and give training for carers in moving and handling, so if you are caring for someone and you have to help them physically, it is worth finding out if this is available near you. This may also be available from other local volunteer organizations.

In some areas you can have smoke alarms and carbon monoxide alarms fitted free if you are elderly and considered to be vulnerable. To find out what is available, it is best to enquire at your local council office or your local public library.

Social life and improving loneliness

Not everyone is naturally outgoing and sociable. However, it is important to well-being and mental alertness to stay in touch with society and to have contact with others on a regular basis. Even if you have difficulty leaving the house due to disability or frailty, this need not prevent you from having social contact. This does not necessarily mean simply meeting people in groups or going to clubs; if you chat regularly to your neighbours, meet others whilst walking the dog or chat to the cashier in the supermarket, this is all 'social contact'. If you belong to any internet chatrooms or communicate through an online forum, this too is social contact.

Social contact is actually therefore hard to avoid. But still, loneliness is a modern problem, with a high percentage of people, especially elderly people, saying that they feel lonely and isolated. A sense of loneliness can often develop following the death of a partner – especially if you have always done things 'as a couple' or following a house move – as your everyday networks change or disappear.

There are some simple ways to improve the amount of contact you have with others and to feel less isolated. It is worth beginning by enlarging on the contacts you have. If you regularly pass the time of day with a neighbour, you could extend that chat by complimenting them on their garden or commenting on their new car. If they go out to work and are always busy, you could offer to take in deliveries for them or to do some other favour so that you get to know them a little better. If you say 'hello' to others when you walk the dog, try chatting to them a little longer next time you see them. Many people testify to the friendships they have made through their pets.

The Silver Line: This registered charity offers advice and information to older people and, in particular, it offers a 'friendship service' via telephone calls. They also offer a service called 'Silver Circles' where people with shared interests can discuss topics that interest them by telephone with a group:

www.thesilverline.org.uk

Volunteering

Many people say that volunteering is a good way to make new friends and to build a social circle. Volunteers are always in demand, although the rules about vetting and training volunteers are much stricter now. This means that many people are put off volunteering at the thought of undergoing security checks and tedious training schedules. However, the amount of training you have to do depends on the volunteer role you take on, so do not be put off without checking first.

Do-it.org is a database of UK volunteering opportunities. You can search what is available in your local area or for your area of interest. There are more than a million volunteering opportunities listed. You can also apply online. The claim is that this is 'volunteering made easy'.

You can also look for opportunities in your specific area by checking with your local council or at your local public library.

Taking part in research

You can volunteer and help yourself, too, by joining the research study, the **PROTECT Study**, being run by the University of Exeter and King's College London in partnership with the NHS. This aims to understand how healthy brains age and why people develop dementia. The study is recruiting people over 50 years old who live in the UK and who do not have a diagnosis of dementia. You do need to be confident using a computer and must have online access to join:

www.protectstudy.org.uk

Health

Many NHS help sites are aimed at people with particular health needs. You can do an online search for any particular health problem. There are also many 'alternative' sites and it can be difficult to decide which advice to trust. One method is to look at whether the particular site or source is advertising a specific product. Sites that advertise are not necessarily untrustworthy, however, as some advertising can help to keep costs down and some charities will accept advertising for this reason. But if a website advertises *only* one particular product, it is worth checking the information against other websites and discussing any advice with a trusted health adviser. Beware, too, of any product that claims to 'cure' medical problems – especially problems that are, at present, considered incurable. Many of such products are harmless and you may like to try them to see if they ease your symptoms, but always check whether the product may react with any medication you are taking. Ask your pharmacist about this as they are very knowledgeable about interactions between drugs and between prescribed medication and 'alternatives'.

Exercise

All research indicates that sensible exercise is good for health and this includes brain health. Many areas have 'Walking for Health' groups to which doctors will sometimes even refer you. In some places doctors will actually give an 'exercise prescription', working with a local gym or sports centre. If you enter your postcode this site will signpost you to Walking for Health groups in your vicinity.

www.walkingforhealth.org.uk

Supported holidays

Many older people with their own health problems are also supporting a partner who needs daily care. Being able to go on holiday can sometimes be very difficult. There are groups that specialize in arranging holidays for older people and that cater for those with physical (and sometimes cognitive) problems. Many of my clients recommend **Warner Leisure Hotels** as giving a good experience without making people feel as if they are set apart from the rest of society:

www.warnerleisurehotels.co.uk

If you and your partner need more specific support, **Revitalise** organize holidays for people with particular care needs including cognitive problems, and they offer activities and excursions on their holidays that include nurse-led care for those who need it:

www.revitalise.org.uk

Remember, too, that most hotels and holiday complexes now have facilities for those who have additional care needs. It is worth enquiring before you book. It can be a pleasant surprise to discover that with a little extra support you can manage a holiday or outing that you thought was not possible.

Living with new technology

Throughout this chapter I have given both website references for many activities and advice an information centres. It is true that many older people find new technology difficult to master, and in most cases you can still obtain information by telephoning or personally enquiring at public libraries, council offices, health centres and similar places. But the information world is moving swiftly, and it can give you a tremendous advantage if you are able to use technology such as smartphones, computers and musical devices. If you do not have dementia, it is almost certain that you can learn to use a technical device even if you think it is beyond you. Of course younger people learn to use technology faster, but there are many ways to learn what you want.

For example, mobile phone shops have trained salespeople who are used to showing older users how to manage their devices and who will take the time to help you. One excellent way to learn the use of any IT device is to ask a younger person to show you how. Grandchildren will often be very happy to show off their knowledge and take pleasure in helping you to understand how to use a phone or an iPad, for example. Many local colleges and centres for education offer courses or workshops to help older people become familiar with new technology.

AbilityNet helps people who are older or disabled to manage new technology and even offers a 'home visit' service. They also offer a number of online support services to help you use a computer:

www.abilitynet.org.uk

Additionally it is worth checking what learning and support services are currently being offered in your area by **Age UK** (see p.199).

I would urge you not to be afraid of new technology but to do your best to master the use of the things that will help you to make your life easier, access information more quickly or get pleasure from your leisure time activities. Bear in mind, too, that if you learn to use something new, you will be helping your brain to develop new pathways and keep cognitive problems at bay.

Key points

- Don't be reluctant to seek help and advice.
- There are many sources of help and advice, and personal support is only one of them.
- Several organizations offer information and advice and most can be accessed by telephone or via the internet as well as by personal contact.
- Not many resources are aimed at MCI generally, but you can look for help on individual topics.
- The internet is a great source of information, but if you prefer, you can use sources such as your local library or local advice centres.
- Don't be afraid of new technology; learn to use it to help yourself or give yourself a better leisure experience.

Endnote

1   See www.citizensadvice.org.uk/about-us/how-we-provide-advice/advice-partnerships/pension-wise

Subject Index